wHoly Fit, wHoly Free

By

Susan Silvestri

wHoly Fit, wHolly Free
Copyright © 2017 by Susan Silvestri
All rights reserved

Published by Silver Settings Press
www.SusanSilvestri.com
"A word fitly spoken is like apples of gold in settings of silver."
Proverbs 25:11

Endorsements

The Fit Tips section of this book is a great guide to showing you ways to maximize your quality of life potential for the rest of your life. The information Susan has provided in the book will serve as inspiration and motivation to live the life that is possible for all of us.

Peter Greenlaw
Author of *Your Third Brain* and
The TDOS Syndrome

Susan Silvestri's new devotional book *wHoly Fit, wHoly Free* is going to ground you in your core, giving you a way to live in strength in the truth of what God has called you to in mind, body, and spirit. She takes her own approach on tying together what has worked so well for her, and she imparts it through a series of prayers, activation activities, Scriptures, and tools to help you. In a very short time, you'll see a significant change and improvement in your life. I believe that, just as if you were taking on a new physical fitness routine, this book will give you the same benefits by the time you are done, but in your very identity.

Shawn Bolz
TV Personality & Author of *Translating God, God Secrets & Growing Up with God*

Sue is such a bright light and true inspiration!

Rachel Boston
Actress, Producer
Hallmark Films

Acknowledgements

Thank you to Heidi Baker for all your love, support and friendship through the years.

Thank you to my editor, Zannie Carlson, who also formatted the book, for your insight, patience and encouragement through the process. I love working with you! (www.zanniecarlson.com)

Thank you to Chris Runco, former Concept Designer at Walt Disney Imagineering, and my Pilates client, for the book cover.

Thank you to Halstan Williams, photographer and director, for your contribution and expert eye on the photos.

Thank you to my brother Tony for your constant support, listening ear, advice, generosity and love. Thanks for the "Island of the Hills" writing haven.

Thank you to Nancy and Derek Lewis for the years of friendship, guidance, hospitality especially during the writing process.

Thank you to Kirk Metz for the support and empowerment of Epic Seasons!

Thank you to Tom Julian, Jul-TV, for the inspiration of planting a seed for a health and fitness devotional.

Thank you to Kingdom Writer's Association (KWA) for inspiring excellence and encouraging vision with fruition.

Thank you to Epiphany Space and my girls at Women of Worth in Hollywood and Expression 58 Lifegroup for being the first ones to open your doors and hearts to the experience of this book!

Dedication

This book is dedicated to my children, Jordan and Karissa Thoma, who inspire me daily to give and live fully and freely. They have taught me sacrifice and unconditional love which has kept my life balanced. Taking care of them even before they were born, contributed to my nutritional perspective of health and wholeness.

They continue to inspire me with their physical strength and discipline and their drive for excellence as Jordan is a stuntman in Hollywood and Karissa is a dancer, choreographer and gymnastics coach. I am proud of them as my children and respect them as people of character and faith. I dedicate this book with love and gratitude to God for them!

Table of Contents

FOREWORD

It is my great joy to write this foreword and highly recommend, *"wHolyFit, wHoly Free,"* by Susan Silvestri. Sue has been a friend of mine for over thirty years. She is in the most incredible physical shape of anyone I know, an awesome dancer who is super fit and healthy, full of vitality and creativity.

I remember when Sue came to Mozambique and danced in our capital city's garbage dump, where I ministered, with as much passion and power as she dances on the stage of any major theater.

I watched her personally take in and care for a severely diseased orphaned child as she gave up her own sleep and comfort to nurture the child back to health and eventually found the little girl an adoptive family.

Sue is a passionate and dedicated woman who cares deeply about God and about health for herself and others. Her heart in writing this book is to encourage and support you as you walk on your journey towards health in your mind, body, soul and spirit.

wHoly Fit, wHoly Free takes you on a forty-day experience towards whole health using Sue's personal experiences, the Bible and the relevant health facts needed to bring you success.

This book gives you tools to choose freedom and health through God's strength, instead of familiar patterns of believing lies about yourself or how God and others may see you. It helps you understand that you are God's beautiful, marvelous creation whom He knows intimately as a Father (Daddy), wanting the very best for you. Sue's passion is to help you, her reader, understand through and through, at a heart and head level, that you have value and worth.

Her book is full of *practical* ways you can build your relationship with God and get to know Him more. Sue speaks truth over you through scripture, poems, and stories. In addition, Sue targets the value of loving yourself through healthy eating and exercise. She cuts through the complexity of most diet plans that can cause guilt and pressure. She gives you easy tips each day that you can put into practice.

wHoly Fit, wHoly Free is not a diet book, but a collection of practical ways to make healthier choices. As Sue writes, **"Instead of dieting the best thing to do is to create a lifestyle change of eating well-balanced, nutritional foods in proper proportion and incorporating some form of exercise."**

When we exercise, dance, or stay active, we feel so much better physically and emotionally. We become stunning women and men shining for God. The goal is to feel healthy and be full of joy and strength. Sometimes it is a huge battle to try and be healthy in our own strength, but when we invite God into each step, the battle becomes much easier. Sue gives powerful tools of journaling, hearing from God, forgiveness, and focusing on God's strength to stay healthy in every area of our lives.

Sue is an extraordinary human being who looks over a decade younger than she is. She is the epitome of health and fitness. I trust her recommendations will be a powerful tool for you and many others to live healthy and whole in God!

Heidi G. Baker, PhD
Co-Founder and CEO of Iris Global

INTRODUCTION

Two women stand next to a scale. One puts her hand out and says, "Don't step on it, it makes you cry."

I've wondered throughout my life, as you may have, if in this world of competition, social media and media in general, it is possible to have a healthy self-image while pursuing excellence. Being in the world of entertainment and performance, as I have been for the past 20 plus years, has only made that question even more relevant. Is it possible to be free in mind and spirit while pursuing being physically fit, or do we have to give up one or the other. After living for years wrestling with these ideas, I can now *weigh in* on them and I've *scaled it down* for you in the following pages!

I have been active most of my life, learning to play many sports at a young age as I tried to keep up with my three brothers while growing up in the Chicago suburbs. My mom put me in dance when I was three years old to keep me from becoming a tomboy. I loved dance and soon excelled in gymnastics as well. At some point, while dancing and competing in track and gymnastics in high school, I realized I could not eat the same as my brothers anymore (two burgers, fries and shake) and still feel good about my looks or performance. So I went on a little diet, for which I received positive feedback and praise from friends and coaches.

After graduating high school, I competed in gymnastics for Northern Illinois University, while getting my BA in Theatre/Dance and Journalism. Our coach had us weigh in almost every day, which encouraged me to diet even more. I felt anxiety stepping onto the scale, along with pressure to have to continue losing weight, even though I was one of the thinnest ones on the team. I was doing gymnastics and dancing seven hours a day and ended up weighing 92 pounds.

One day, I woke up so hungry that I couldn't eat. Food had become the enemy. I fought a war in my mind and spirit with a distorted view of myself and nutrition until a few years after I had graduated and married. I was still trying to maintain my identity and value, to some degree, through being thin during the daily rigors of owning a gymnastics academy, coaching top level gymnasts, dancing in a company, and being a new bride. But something amazing happened when I got pregnant with my son. It was then my mind shifted to food no longer being evil but something positive to sustain and nourish a life that was being formed in me.

After my son was born, I came to the realization that I needed to treat myself with the same respect and love I did when I was caring for him in the womb. That could only come from understanding my value to God and myself, understanding that the motive for keeping a healthy body was to operate at my best for all I was meant to do and be.

My significance was not based on my performance or appearance.

I have been a professional dancer and actor in film and on stage for over twenty years so I know what it is like to persevere in trying to keep a healthy self-perception through the pressures of performance and competition. I have also tried to impart that truth into those I have worked with as I coached national champion gymnasts for years and am a certified Pilates instructor.

In my quest to be physically fit and function at my highest level, I have had to learn to be holistically healthy.

FIT and FREE in my mind, body, soul and spirit.

I have tried to educate myself about all aspects of nutrition. I have had to learn to fight battles of perfectionism, fear, comparison, guilt, and self-condemnation by replacing lies with the truth of the way God sees me.

God thinks I am beautifully and wonderfully made!

He thinks that about you, too!

And He wants us to love and value ourselves and others by understanding how He sees us. Once we grasp how much He loves and delights in us as His precious children, nutritional discipline and perseverance become a joy. Our motivation turns from pressuring ourselves for perfection to *choosing* to take care of ourselves because of the abundant blessings that operating at our fullest potential provide.

Hopefully, this book will help and encourage you to connect to the truth and beauty within yourself, to see yourself through God's eyes, and to give you inspired vision for all God has for you.

"May God himself, the God who makes everything holy and whole, put you together - spirit, soul and body - and keep you fit..."
I Thessalonians 5:23 (The Message)

Susan Silvestri
Author, wHoly Fit, wHoly Free

wHoly Fit, wHoly Free

To be wholly who you are designed to be is to be fit and free in mind, body, soul and spirit. When all four are working together and are in alignment, a balance is created that allows you to be the best YOU possible. Just as in Pilates, it all starts at the core, which empowers everything else.

In this case the core is **value**.

If you really desire to live a fulfilled life, you must first believe that you are worthy of it. You are valuable to God and the world around you and are worthy of love and respect from yourself, God and others.

God created you as unique and His original design for you is not to be perfect, but to be the best version of you that you can be.

"You formed my inward parts;
You covered me in my mother's womb.
My frame was not hidden from You,
When I was made in secret,
And skillfully wrought."

Psalm 139:13,15 (NKJV)

The creator of the universe who created two to fifty million different types of species, created YOU with the unique differences that make you beautiful and special.

Instead of comparing yourself to others or striving to be like what the media promotes, you can shift your mind to celebrate the things that set you apart and highlight your special qualities, believing the Master Potter has designed you with a specific idea in mind. He didn't forget or leave anything out, nor did He add something that didn't need to be there. He was intentional about how He formed you and wants to give the world a unique and individual aspect of His character through you.

When you transform your perspective, you begin seeing what you think are *flaws* or *faults* in your physical form as highlighted unique qualities that help make you an original design. As you transform your mind and see yourself as unique and valuable, it will help kick start the motivation and give you a vision for transforming your body through nutrition and fitness. In turn, healthy eating and exercise help generate your brain function and give you physical energy, creating endorphins that help calm your heart and bring joy to your soul.

When you're feeling good about yourself and are at peace, it is easier to receive love from God and others. Likewise, when your spirit is being fed and you know you're cherished unconditionally by a loving Father, it releases you, freeing you to want to live up to your fullest potential. It empowers you to walk in the significance and destiny God has created you for. It gives you vision for a life full of purpose and impact. It's no longer a burden, but a privilege to take care of yourself. It's not a bondage of rules and religion, but a roadmap to freedom for relationship with yourself, God and others.

I want to help direct you on that path. This book is not meant to be a diet or nutrition plan book per se, but is mostly to inspire and help set habits and perspective, not only physically but mentally, emotionally and spiritually.

It is a 40 day/40 way journey to wholeness.

Each daily reading has an inspirational verse to meditate on for your spirit, food for thought for your mind, an activational journaling prompt for your heart and soul, and a "Fit Tip", nutrition or exercise idea for your body.

I want you to see this devotional as not just a book of information, but an invitation to participate in transforming your mind, body, soul and spirit to be all you were created to be.

JOURNALING

Journaling can be more than just writing your thoughts, feelings or events from the day. It can be an active conversation.

I've enjoyed journaling ever since I can remember. I was given a diary for Christmas in fourth grade and would diligently write every day, which helped me process thoughts and feelings in a way I couldn't do with friends or family. Being the only girl with three brothers, I felt a bit lonely or misunderstood at times. By the time Junior High rolled around, I started using spiral notebooks to write in as I went through them quite quickly. Teen years can require many pages!

My notebook became like a special friend to me; one I could share secrets with. I went from "Dear Diary" to "Dear Sunny" and then sometime around High School, "Dear God", as I grew to know Him.

Fast forward - years, tears, fears, cheers, careers later...

I discovered a new form of journaling where it was two-way. I was no longer just expressing my heart, but learning to get wisdom and understanding by hearing the voice of God for my life through journaling. It became a conversation with listening and not just a monologue of speaking.

Everyone is hungry for a word of hope for his/her life. Some people go to a psychic or palm reader. Christians wait for a prophetic word from a preacher or a friend in prayer.

The truth is you can be receiving these words every day for yourself.

God wants to speak words of truth, hope and life into you to renew and transform your mind, revive and strengthen your body, restore and love your soul, and refresh and empower your spirit. He is all about relationship and conversation.

"Come now, and let us reason together, says the Lord."

Isaiah 1:18 (NASB)

The "Activate" sections of this book are meant to prompt and inspire you to participate in hearing this voice of wisdom and truth for yourself through journaling. According to Mark Virkler, founder of Communion with God Ministries, there are four keys to unlocking the door to hearing the voice of God through this two-way journaling.

Key One: Get in a quiet place and still your thoughts and emotions. Remove yourself from distraction and put on some soft music or music that inspires you.

Key Two: Visualize yourself in one of your favorite places. Maybe a peaceful place, like the beach, or a big green field, or the mountains. Picture God being there with you.

"Come near to God and he will come near to you."

James 4:8 (NIV)

Ask Him a question like, "What are your thoughts toward me?" or "Do you love me?" (There are different questions you will be asking in the activations.)

22

Key Three:	Wait for God's still small voice.

> *"I pray that the eyes of your heart may be enlightened in order that you may know the hope to which he has called you."*

> *Ephesians 1:18 (NIV)*

A great story about a man who heard God's voice is found in the book of I Kings. Elijah was running away from his circumstances in much fear, when an angel led him to a place where he waited to hear from God. He looked for God to speak to him in a great and powerful wind, in an earthquake and in fire. It was not in any of these that God spoke. It was in a still, small voice, like a whisper. (I Kings 19:12). That was the way God told him what his next step was. God's voice usually comes as spontaneous thoughts, visions, feelings, or impressions. Wait for the flow of free thoughts to come in answer to your question.

Key Four:	Write what you hear in the still, small voice. Don't edit it or question it until you're done. Just write…

> *"I will stand my watch and set myself on the rampart, and watch to see what He will say to me…The Lord answered me and said: 'Write the vision and make it plain on tablets, that he may run who reads it. For the vision is yet for an appointed time; But at the end it will speak, and it will not lie. Though it tarries, wait for it; because it will surely come, it will not tarry.'"*

> *Habakkuk 2:1-3 (NKJV)*

You can test it after you're done. You will know if it's God's voice if it lines up with His character and Word. He speaks truth, love, mercy, grace, peace, kindness, goodness. He does not condemn or bring confusion. He speaks life, encouragement, and hope. It may come in a style that you don't normally write in. God is creative in communicating to us.

Prophecy is basically speaking God's heart of love (His truth and will) for someone. Two-way journaling is learning how to hear God's heart, or prophetic word, for yourself.

Simply quiet yourself down, tune to spontaneity, look for vision, and journal. It's exciting to see what can be revealed!

*You can find out more about Mark's teaching under the Recommended Reading section in the back of the book.

PART ONE

MIND

MIND

The mind is described as the part of a person that thinks, reasons, feels, perceives, and remembers. Everything starts in the mind. It's what gives vision to your life and goals. It also directs your actions and your heart.

"For as he THINKS in his heart, so is he."

Proverbs 23:7 (AMP)

The mind affects your perception of yourself. This is known as self-image, or the way you imagine yourself to be. When you transform your mind to stay fixed on what God says about you and how He sees you, then you can more easily fight the false perceptions and the lies put on you by the world, others or yourself, and stand in the truth of who you were created to be.

Once you get a clear self-perception and are able to focus your mind positively on "whatever is true, whatever is noble, whatever is right, whatever is pure, whatever is lovely, whatever is admirable...excellent or praiseworthy" Philippians 4:8 (NIV), then getting fit takes on a whole new perspective. It becomes a joy, not drudgery. There is freedom in it.

Becoming fit and free starts in the mind, which sets the course for wholeness.

MIND

Your mind holds you captive
Or your mind sets you free
Depending on the insight
You set your thoughts to see.
Reclaiming your self-image
Breaking the world of lies
As you look in the mirror
Seeing through God's eyes.
You can know the truth
And it will set you free
To be the fullest person
You were meant to be.
Your mind is renewed daily
With what you believe
Transforming your whole being
From what you perceive.
Not dwelling on earthly things
Set your mind on things above
And you'll live without fear
In the soundness of God's love.
Focusing on what is noble
Admirable, right and true
You will begin to activate
The best version of you.
What's excellent and lovely
Think on all these things
And you'll experience peace
And wholeness that it brings.

Day 1

YOUR REFLECTION

Inspiration

"For now we see only a reflection as in a mirror; then we shall see face to face. Now I know in part; then I shall know fully, even as I am fully known."

I Corinthians 13:12 (NIV)

Food for Thought

Often times you look in the mirror and see only your flaws or distorted versions of who you really are. Someone with anorexia can look in the mirror and will actually see her/himself ten to twenty pounds heavier. In order to see who you really are, you have to be able to see yourself through the eyes of the One who created you.

When this verse was written, mirrors were made in Corinth with metal and only gave dim reflections. Nowadays, looking glasses give very clear reflections, but the verse still holds true because many people see a distortion of the truth in the mirror. You may look in the mirror and see someone whose nose is too big or who is too fat or whose figure isn't perfect. You are seeing dimly. You will begin to see yourself more clearly when you go face to face with God. When you look to Him to see your reflection through His eyes, you can know the truth of who you really are.

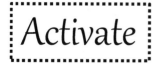

Activate

Look at yourself in the mirror and write down what you see. Then close your eyes and picture God face to face with you. Ask Him what He sees. Open your eyes and look in the mirror again. Now write what you see through His eyes for you.

Thoughts

_____

_____

_____

_____

_____

_____

_____

_____

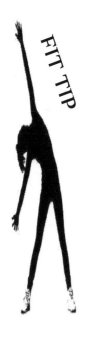

FIT TIP

Go nuts for brain health!

It's interesting that the walnut looks like a mini version of your brain and happens to be high in in omega-3 fatty acids and protein, which makes it a healthy brain wave food. Nuts, in general, can also be a good source of magnesium, vitamin E, fiber and other nutrients that can actually boost metabolism and curb appetite.

A handful of nuts makes a healthful snack.

Did you know that it's believed that you actually have more than one brain? Your "first brain", located in the head (sometimes referred to as your "nut") is an organ that serves as the center of the nervous system. You'll be enlightened about your "second brain" on Day 2.

Day 2

GOD'S THOUGHTS TOWARD YOU

Inspiration

"You have searched me, Lord, and you know me. You know when I sit and when I rise: you perceive my thoughts from afar. You discern my going out and my lying down; you are familiar with all my ways. Before a word is on my tongue you, Lord, know it completely. You hem me in behind and before, and you lay your hand upon me. Such knowledge is too wonderful for me ...

All the days ordained for me were written in your book before one of them came to be. How precious to me are your thoughts God! How vast is the sum of them! Were I to count them, they would outnumber the grains of sand."

Psalm 139:1-6, 16-18. (NIV)

Food for Thought

Everyone desires to be known. To have someone understand their thoughts and mind in a way that goes beyond themselves. Unfortunately, too often people may look to another person to fill this deep longing. God is the one who holds the key to filling it. Not only does He know you intimately, but He knew all your days before they came to be. Nothing surprises Him or turns Him away. The Creator of the Universe thinks about you personally all the time! His thoughts toward you are immeasurable. They are more than the grains of sand. He is constantly thinking about you.

Activate

Get in a quiet place. Picture yourself in one of your favorite spaces - maybe on the beach or in a big green field. Now picture God with you, walking or sitting by your side. Ask Him what His thoughts toward you are. Wait until you hear a still, small voice or have a spontaneous thought or impression. Write down whatever comes to you. Let it flow on the page without editing it as God gives you His mind for you.

_____

_____

_____

_____

_____

_____

_____

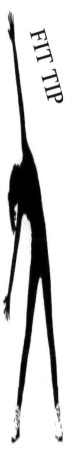

FIT TIP

Healthy gut, healthy nut!

To have a healthy nut (first brain), you need a healthy gut (second brain). Your 'second brain' is believed to be in the lining of your gut or gastrointestinal tract. It contains as many neurons as in the first brain - some 100 million. This network of neurons lining the digestive tract is what causes that nervous pit in your stomach known as 'butterflies', which are stress responders. 90 percent of the cells carry information to the first brain, so when your gut is healthy, it affects clarity of your mind and mood. That's why many psychiatrists are now treating mental challenges first in the gut, with much success.

This is good news for those who suffer from anxiety or depression. There is evidence that a healthy gut can curb inflammation and cortisol levels, lower your reaction to stress, improve memory and even reduce neuroticism and social anxiety.

It is often recommended to stay away from hard-to-digest gluten in wheat products and casein in pasteurized milk products. Doing this can actually help with focus of the brain and has been associated with dramatically relieving symptoms of ADHD and Parkinson's.

There are more tips on how to maintain a healthy gut throughout the book. You can also go to www.SusanSilvestri.com for personalized solutions.

TAKE CAPTIVE EVERY THOUGHT

Inspiration

"The weapons we fight with are not the weapons of the world. On the contrary, they have divine power to demolish strongholds. We demolish arguments and every pretension that sets itself up against the knowledge of God, and we take captive every thought."

2 Corinthians 10:5 (NIV)

Food for Thought

In order to have a healthy mind, you need to get rid of the thoughts that go against who God says you are or who He is. These thoughts are the arguments and every pretension that put themselves above the knowledge of God. In other words, they're vain imaginations, or falsehoods, that get magnified in your mind to appear as truths or appear larger than they are. These thoughts create strongholds that keep you in bondage. Strongholds are lies based out of fear and not trusting in God's provision and in the knowledge of who He really is.

You have the power to demolish these strongholds by taking hold of these thoughts, recognizing them, and replacing them with the truth of who God is and all He has done to free you from these bondages of the mind. Jesus put to death those strongholds on the cross so you could live in this resurrection power.

Activate

Is there a stronghold in your life that keeps you in bondage? Ask God if there's a lie you are believing that keeps you there. What is the fear behind it? For instance, maybe you are in bondage to the constant thoughts of losing weight and guilt for eating. Your fear may be that people won't like you if you're not perfect or thin. Write down what God shows you.

Next to the lie write the truth. Cross out the lie and release it into God's hands as you trust Him to demolish the stronghold (lie that you've believed about yourself) and replace it with truth.

Thoughts

_____

_____

_____

When your gut is healthy and fit, the rest of your organs feel it!

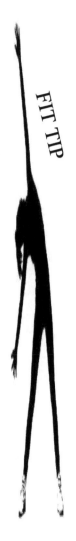

The "second brain", or the gut, is believed to also be responsible for all other organs from your brain to your immune system.

The bacteria in the gut flora communicate with the important neurotransmitters embedded throughout the body which are called the microbiome. You have as many microbiome as your own human cells. According to Dr. Marco Ruggiero and Peter Greenlaw, authors of *Your Third Brain*, the microbiome is the complex organ considered your "third brain".

The gut bacteria affecting the microbiome has been with you since birth, helping digest food and fight off viruses and molds. Unfortunately, things such as antibiotics can kill good bacteria. In order to promote the growth of beneficial gut bacteria, while helping crowd out and eliminate harmful bacteria causing inflammation from unhealthy foods, you need probiotics and prebiotics.

Probiotics (living, friendly bacteria) are naturally found in cultured or fermented foods, such as yogurt (with lactobacillus, acidophilus), kefir, buttermilk, aged cheese, sauerkraut, kimchi, miso, and kombucha, a type of fermented tea. They can also be taken in supplement form.

Be careful when labels say "probiotic benefits", such as on certain yogurts. Because of the pasteurization process, there may be little to no benefit and, depending on the sugar or high fructose corn syrup content, may be more harmful than good. Sugar feeds candida (bad bacteria in the gut), which causes bloating. Always read labels.

Prebiotics (non-living food ingredients) go straight to the large intestine unaffected by digestion and "feed" the good bacteria in your gut, helping them to grow and flourish. They are naturally found in many foods, including garlic, artichokes, cabbage, legumes, and onions.

A good protein shake with prebiotic is listed under Recommended Resources in the back of the book. (1)

FIT TIP

Day 4

SOUND MIND

"For God has not given us a spirit of fear, but of power and of love and of a sound mind."

2 Timothy 1:7 (NKJV)

Food for Thought

Having a sound mind literally means "safe-thinking" in the Greek ("sophronismos"). It includes good judgment, disciplined thought patterns, and the ability to understand and make right decisions, including having self-control and self-discipline.

One of the things that keeps you from having a sound mind is fear. Another word for fear is timidity. This can make you feel powerless and alone. It can hold you back from what you are meant to do. It can make you indecisive or influence you to make wrong decisions, which can put you in bondage. Your fullness and freedom is found in plugging into the power source of the Holy Spirit and the love and the mind of God. (Philippians 2:5).

41

Activate

Is there anything in particular that you are fearful or indecisive about that is keeping you from having a sound mind or self-discipline? Is there anything that seems to be keeping you from being all you were created for? Maybe you're afraid you will not be able to live up to the expectations you put on yourself.

Ask God to show you what that fear or those fears might be and how His power and love can overcome them to bring you to a place of safe thinking. Write what He reveals.

Thoughts

_____

_____

_____

_____

_____

_____

_____

_____

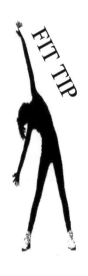

FIT TIP

Keep your mind sane with a walk up memory lane!

Regular exercise, including walking, increases memory. A Harvard study showed that 120 minutes of moderate intensity exercise per week can improve memory. This can be an hour of brisk walking twice a week or even doing household chores that get your heart rate up. You can break it down to 20-30 minutes a day, but if even that seems overwhelming, just start with walking ten minutes around the block.

Something is always better than nothing!

Day 5

MIND ON THINGS ABOVE

Inspiration

"Set your minds on things above, not on earthly things."

Colossians 3:2 (NIV)

"But the LORD said to Samuel, 'Don't judge by his appearance or height.... The LORD doesn't see things the way you see them. People judge by outward appearance, but the LORD looks at the heart.'"

I Samuel 16:7 (NLT)

Food for Thought

What are the "things above"? They are the way God sees you and the way He sees the world through a timeless eternal lens. The invisible realm as opposed to the material world. His perspective as opposed to the world's perspective. When you set your mind to see through His eyes, a whole new world is opened to you. Somehow, you become less consumed or worried about what others think of you. You see yourself according to the way God sees you, which gives you self-confidence. Focusing on the things above helps you look outward instead of inward and to become more aware of the hurting people around you.

Society tries to put an image on you of how you are supposed to look through the media. It glorifies overly skinny young women or perfectly chiseled men, while demonizing weight or wrinkles. The messages we receive through television, movies and social media focus more on outward appearance than inward beauty or character. When you measure yourself according to this standard, you put yourself in bondage and judge yourself and others accordingly. God looks at the heart. When you set your mind on the things above, which are the total person - mind, body, soul, spirit - then the burden of having to live up to a false image is replaced with the freedom of seeing yourself for the whole person you really are.

Activate

Write down the image or look you feel pressured by the world to have. Write a list of characteristics. Now write a list of the "things above" - the inner qualities of the heart that you possess. Ask God to show you - He may highlight things you didn't even realize you had in yourself. Ask God to help you let go of the first list and set your mind on the strengths He's shown you.

Thoughts

_____

_____

_____

Strengthen your mind with muscle.

Strength training is not just for outward results, but can benefit you intrinsically including in your mind. Strength training can boost your long term memory and lower your risk of dementia. Researchers at Georgia Institute of Technology in Atlanta found that a mere twenty minute weight training session could improve long-term memory.

Strength training is a way to increase lean body mass, decrease fat mass, and increase resting metabolic rate, better known as metabolism (a measurement of the amount of calories burned per day), in adults. Strength training regularly helps preserve lean muscle tissue and can even rebuild what's been lost already. A healthy lifestyle will support your brain health, and can even encourage your brain to grow new neurons—a process known as *neurogenesis* or *neuroplasticity*.

The training doesn't have to be in a gym with machines. You can strength train simply by doing push-ups and sit-ups at home, using your own body weight for resistance. Just ten push-ups and fifty sit-ups twice or three times a week can help maintain muscle. You can also do it by carrying heavy loads (with proper posture, using your core) or doing things like heavy gardening.

FIT TIP

Day 6

RENEWING YOUR MIND

Inspiration

"Do not conform to the pattern of this world, but be transformed by the renewing of your mind. Then you will be able to test and approve what God's will is--His good, pleasing and perfect will."

Romans 12:2 (NIV)

"For I know the plans I have for you," declares the Lord, "plans to prosper you and not to harm you, plans to give you hope and a future.

Jeremiah 29:11 (NIV)

Food for Thought

You are transformed by renewing your mind. To renew is to restore or renovate. When you renew your mind, you refresh or restore it to its original state. In other words, you set your mind on the created intent, plans God has, for your life.

God had a plan for you with purpose and significance from the beginning. It's easy to get lost in the pattern of this world, thinking you don't match up or are not "perfect" enough. You can feel disqualified or insignificant. He doesn't ask us to be perfect but to live in the place that is good and pleasing. His perfect will for you is that you be the best version of you. He has a purpose and plan for your life that is unique in the world that only you can fulfill. His good, pleasing and perfect will is for you to live in your value, understanding the fullness of your worth and knowing you have a future and a hope.

Activate

Ask God what He created you for. Is there an area of your life where you have lost hope or vision? Ask God to renew that and give you a vision for your future. Record the vision! (Habakkuk 2:2)

Thoughts

_____

_____

_____

_____

_____

_____

_____

_____

_____

_____

_____

_____

_____

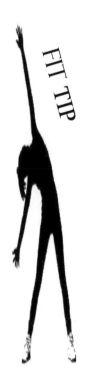

FIT TIP

Vision foods have colorful hues!

Foods that are good for vision include carrots and other orange fruits and vegetables because of the beta-carotene they contain, which is a type of vitamin A that gives these foods their orange hue. They help the retina and other parts of the eye to function smoothly. Leafy greens and yellow egg yolks have lutein and zeaxanthin, antioxidants that lower the risk of developing macular degeneration and cataracts. Colorful citrus and berries with high doses of vitamin C help with that as well.

On the more neutral side of the color chart, besides being good brain food, a handful of almonds contains half the daily dose of vitamin E needed for healthy eyesight. Fatty fish, such as tuna, salmon, mackerel, anchovies and trout are rich in DHA, a fatty acid found in your retina. Low levels of this can cause dry eye syndrome.

"Holy Mackerel" - 1 can see!

Day 7

POSITIVE THOUGHTS

Inspiration

"...whatever is true, whatever is noble, whatever is right, whatever is pure, whatever is lovely, whatever is admirable – if anything is excellent or praiseworthy – think about such things."

Philippians 4:8 (NIV)

Food for Thought

What is something about yourself that is true, that is noble, that is right, that is pure, lovely, admirable, excellent, praiseworthy?

This is a good checklist to use to keep a healthy mind. Your biggest warfare, or battle, takes place in your mind. There is a constant struggle between lies and truth, light and dark, negative and positive, God's voice and the enemy's voice. God's voice always lines up with His character of love and peace; He doesn't condemn or accuse.

When you choose to focus your mind on these qualities, the lies dissipate, leaving no room for the negative because the truth shines through. It's like a light in the darkness. When you turn on the light, it overpowers the darkness.

When negative thoughts come into your mind, especially about yourself, like, "I'm too fat, I'm not attractive, I'm not loved" check them against the Philippians verse. Are they true, noble, right, etc? Dispel the lie, with the truth.

Use this list to measure your thoughts towards others and circumstances as well.

Activate

Write down the eight positive words that Philippians 4:8 tells you to think about. Next to each one, write down something about yourself that correlates with it - something true, noble, right, pure, lovely, admirable, excellent, and praiseworthy. Find synonyms for these words if it helps, such as "sincere" or "authentic" for "true" or "honorable" for "noble."

Ask God what He sees in you for each word.

Thoughts

_____

_____

_____

_____

_____

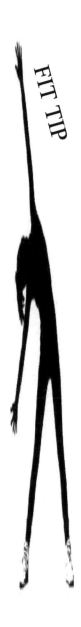

Protein can help boost positivity!

Eating good sources of protein helps to boost our levels of **serotonin** and **dopamine** and this is really important, as these help to boost energy, and mental clarity, and basically make you feel happier. They also regulate pain, reduce anxiety, and initiate deep sleep.

A morning meal that's rich in protein can also help you lose weight by keeping you full, satisfied and less likely to overeat. If you eat protein within a half hour of waking up, it can jump-start your metabolism.

It's important to look for proteins that have a high Net Protein Utilization (NPU). This is the amount of protein that's absorbed into the bloodstream. Some protein foods actually have very low NPU because of the way they are broken down in the body. A couple of foods that have high percentage of NPU are eggs and whey. There is a good undenatured (unaltered, natural) whey protein recommended in the back of the book that has 97% NPU. (1)

Proteins in our diet affect brain performance because they provide the amino acids that make up our neurotransmitters - biochemical messengers whose job it is to carry signals from one brain cell to another.

As you eat more protein, you may find you strengthen not only your body, but your peace of mind!

Day 8

PERCEPTION

*"You will be a crown of splendor in the Lord's hand,
a royal diadem in the hand of your God."*

Isaiah 62:3 (NIV)

*"Because you are precious in my eyes, and honored, and I love
you"*

Isaiah 43:4 (ESV)

:::
: Food for Thought :
:::

Often because of a negative church experience or other
circumstances, you may have a false perception of who you are to
God, which, in turn, causes you to have a negative perception of
yourself. In reality, God knows your faults but your beauty
outshines them; He knows all you have been through, which is
actually what He uses to make you the gem that you
are. Adversity can create the resistance needed to mold you into
the precious stone, just like most natural diamonds are formed at
high temperatures and with great pressure, deep under the earth's
surface. In the same way, an oyster protects itself from the constant
irritation of an intruder (like a piece of sand) by forming a

protective covering called nacre (mother of pearl). The irritations in your life are what are forming you and making you shine, if you allow God to work through them and be the protective covering.

Jesus spoke in parables about the "pearl of great price". He likened it to His Kingdom and since you are part of it, YOU are a pearl of great price! He calls you a "crown of splendor (beauty) and a royal diadem (gem)." He sees all and knows you even better than you know yourself and yet sees the royal version of you because you are His princess/prince. Keep in mind, the more rare the gem, the more valuable!

Activate

Look at a gorgeous gem you may have or may be wearing - maybe a diamond or pearl. Examine the beauty of it. Think of God looking at you the way you are looking at the stone. Ask Him and write down what He sees in you. What kind of gem would you be? What color?

Thoughts

_____

_____

_____

_____

_____

_____

_____

_____

_____

_____

_____

_____

_____

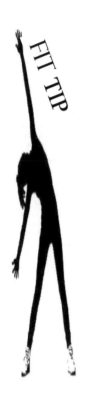

Something's "fishy"!!

Mental clarity can help with perception. Certain foods can increase mental alertness and cognitive function. Many of the same foods that help with vision clarity can also be beneficial for mental clarity. Fish, such as salmon, trout, mackerel, and sardines, have the essential fatty acids and Omega 3 for mental clarity to help manage stress and improve mood from the brain chemical serotonin. Blueberries and blackberries have antioxidants that can help reverse age-related memory loss. Spinach and other dark leafy greens have folate and vitamin E and K that can boost memory. Egg yolks contain choline which is associated with improved mental alertness and memory. Green tea and dark chocolate (at least 72 percent) are also beneficial brain boosters.

Day 9

KNOWING YOUR IDENTITY

Inspiration

"'I will be a Father to you, and you will be my sons and daughters,'
says the Lord Almighty."

2 Corinthians 6:17-18 (NIV)

"How great is the love the Father has lavished on us, that we
should be called children of God! And that is what we are!"

1 John 3:1 (NIV)

Food for Thought

The first question people usually ask when they meet you is
"What do you do?" Actors are asked "What have you done?" A
business person's worth is judged by his/her resume. Your identity
is not in *what you do* but in *who you are*, or rather *whose* you are!
You are a child of God, the creator of the universe and the one
who knows every hair on your head!

He is a loving Father. You may not have grown up with an earthly father who treated you with the value that you deserved, but God's love is unconditional for His children. He is protective, personal and passionate about your well-being. When you really know who you are you can stand securely in your identity, knowing your Heavenly Father will take care of you and you can proclaim your true inheritance which He has promised you as a child of God.

Activate

Ask God to reveal Himself to you as a loving Father. What would a loving father look like? If there is anything in the way of that, ask Him to show you and invite Him to be the protector of your heart, provider of your well-being and the loving Father you desire.

Thoughts

_____

_____

_____

_____

_____

_____

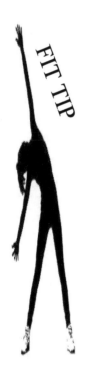

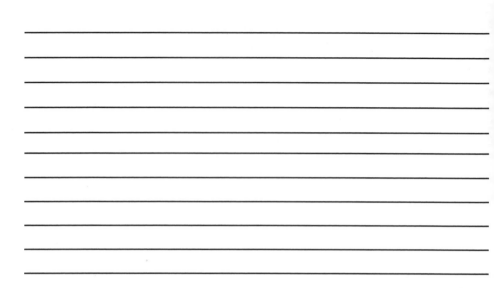

Memory identity!

Supplements such as ginkgo biloba can be taken to help boost memory. Green Tea is another effective brain health enhancer. Turmeric is also known for its properties of promoting mental health along with other healing benefits. It's even been theorized that the gold brought by one of the three Wisemen was actually turmeric because it was a gold colored treasure of healing and health from the East.

Gingko biloba, green tea and turmeric together are especially effective in increasing mental focus, concentration, decision-making and memory. There is a supplement with this combination recommended in the back of the book. (2)

Day 10

KNOWING TRUTH BRINGS FREEDOM

Inspiration

*"And you shall know the truth, and the truth shall make you free...
Therefore, if the Son makes you free you shall be free indeed."*

John 8:32 (AMP)

*"For God so [greatly] loved and dearly prized the world
(YOU), that He [even] gave His [One and] only begotten Son, so
that whoever believes and trusts in Him [as Savior] shall not
perish, but have eternal life."*

John 3:16 (AMP)

Food for Thought

You've probably heard the phrase "knowledge is power" taken
from the Latin aphorism "Scientia potentia est". When you know
the truth, it has power to set you free.

These verses state that God loves you so much that He sent His
Son to be a sacrifice for you so that anything that holds you back

from being all you were created to be can be buried. You can have resurrection power to set you free to live fully.

Knowing the truth of who you are and who God created you to be and who you are in Him, sets you free to be all you are meant to be. If you live in the truth of how much Jesus loves you and what He paid for you and your freedom, you will be truly free to move in the fullness of all that He has for you.

Activate

Ask God what are some truths about yourself according to God's Word and His love for you. Now express His love through you or to you by writing, or drawing, or dancing. Maybe put on a song such as *How He Loves Us (Kim Walker) or Reckless Love (Cory Asbury)*. Turn knowledge of His truth and love for you into freedom for your life.

Thoughts

_____

_____

_____

_____

_____

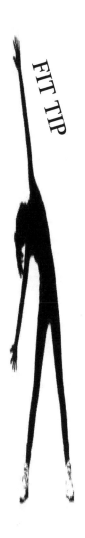

FIT TIP

Dance your way to freedom and health!

Dancing is freedom of expression, freedom from depression, and a risk reduction! Frequent dancing can ward off Alzheimer's disease and other dementia, according to a study in The New England Journal of Medicine. There is a 76% risk reduction for these diseases because dancing integrates several brain functions at once - kinesthetic, rational, musical, and emotional - further increasing your neural connectivity by blending cerebral and cognitive thought processes with muscle memory and body awareness held in the cerebellum. No wonder dance has been a social exercise in just about every culture throughout history!

Dance, along with other aerobic exercise, can reverse volume loss in the hippocampus, the part of the brain that controls memory. The hippocampus naturally shrinks during late adulthood, which often leads to impaired memory and sometimes dementia, but dancing can keep you young in mind and spirit!

PART TWO
BODY

BODY

Your body is the outward representation of the inward you. It is defined as the structure of a human organism. It's your flesh as opposed to spirit; tangible as opposed to incorporeal. When your body is operating at its full potential, you are more apt to have a healthy mindset and vibrant spirit. Nutrition and exercise help to keep your body, or "temple", in order and fit. This, in turn, frees you to do physical activities. Sometimes you need to remove the pressure to be perfect and allow God to give you the discipline and joy to help in this process. You were created to use your body for more than just outward appearance. Your body functions as an instrument to not only accomplish tasks, but to be a display of splendor, an expression of praise and glory.

That means that no matter where you are fit- or weight-wise, you can be like David and use your body as an expression of joy, surrendering fully - even the feeling of imperfection. Loving and respecting your body, no matter how you may feel about it, is another form of worship.

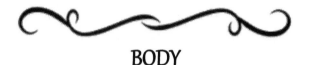

BODY

Your body is a vessel
An instrument of His story
Outwardly displaying splendor
Inward beauty of God's glory.
It's like a magnificent temple
An entrusted, honored shrine
Fulfilling His heart's intent
To let your true light shine.
The discipline of the body
Plays an important part
But where it all originates
Is discipline of the heart.
Don't put yourself under law
To keep it perfect and clean
The Spirit gives you strength
To keep it mean and lean.
You were made for freedom
So let your inhibition go
David danced unreservedly
So let your movement flow.
In God you live and breathe
And have your very being.
You see outward appearance
Your heart is what He's seeing.

Skillfully crafted and wrought
From timeless foundation laid.
Designed in your mother's womb
Fearfully and wonderfully made.
Trust Him to make you strong
He'll give you what you lack
Trust Him in ALL your ways
And He will direct your path.
Making imperfections perfect
Making crooked ways straight
He gets you back on track
With Him it's never too late.
No matter where you're at
You're beautiful in His sight
The strength is by His Spirit
Not by your power or might.
Surrendering your human flesh
Your will power and diet plans
He can lead you on the journey
Your whole body in His hands.
Running the race set before you
With the goal of God's treasure
Striding toward the finish mark
You will surely feel His pleasure.

Day 11

WONDERFULLY MADE

"You created my inmost being; you knit me together in my mother's womb. I praise you because I am fearfully and wonderfully made; your works are wonderful, I know that full well. My frame was not hidden from you when I was made in the secret place, when I was woven together in the depths of the earth. Your eyes saw my unformed body."

Psalm 139: 13-16 (NIV)

Food for Thought

God made you just the way you are. He didn't make a mistake in forming you. You were specially designed. The Hebrew word for "wonderful" is *pil'iy*, meaning beyond human perception, requiring supernatural insight in order to be able to see. It takes seeing yourself through God's eyes in order to be able to see who you really are and to understand how special you are.

The Young's Literal Translation says "with wonders I have been distinguished." You were designed specifically by the Master

75

Designer. He *distinguished* you from others, perhaps with a prominent attribute. People tend to see their distinctive features as physical flaws instead of God's creativity in making them unique. God had something specific in mind when He formed you. The more you thank God for the way He created you and see His amazing handiwork, the more at peace with yourself you will be.

Activate

Picture God crafting you while He was forming you in your mother's womb, like a sculptor making you precisely and uniquely the way He designed - every detail. Picture Him carving, molding even the areas you struggle with. Is there something about your body that you don't particularly like? Ask Him to show you the beauty and uniqueness in that - in who you are and how you were formed.

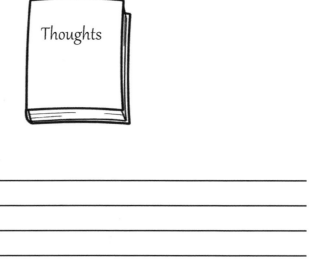

Thoughts

_____

_____

_____

_____

_____

_____

_____

_____

_____

_____

_____

_____

_____

_____

_____

_____

_____

_____

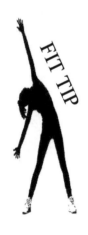

Counting your calories as blessings!

If you want to know how many calories a day you should eat, take your ideal body weight and add a "0" to the end. If it is 125 lbs., then you should eat at least 1250 calories a day in 4 to 6 meals. If you work out add 300-500 calories.

A simple way to measure nourishment for your day!

Day 12

FREEDOM TO CHOOSE

Inspiration

"All things are lawful for me, but all things are not helpful. All things are lawful for me, but I will not be brought under the power of any... For you were bought at a price; therefore glorify God in your body and in your spirit, which are God's."

I Corinthians 6:12 (NKJV)

Food for Thought

God gives you the freedom to choose as far as your bodies are concerned. You are not under law or condemnation - He wants you to choose what is *helpful* in bringing you to your full potential in all He has designed you for and what draws you closer to His heart. The price He paid was for you to be able to have relationship with Him and live in His love and fullness. He simply wants you to choose that path.

When you look to what's helpful in bringing you closer to Him and the plans He has for you, then you can choose to walk in the freedom of not letting anything have power over you.

Sometimes you may put yourself under the law of a strict diet plan and then when you don't follow through with it you condemn yourself. If you take the approach that all things are lawful (permissible) but not helpful (best), you then do it not out of being imprisoned to it, but because there is a higher purpose. That frees you from being under the control of it.

Activate

Is there anything that holds you back or is not helpful in you being the best person you can be? Maybe it's an addiction. Or maybe it's a trap in your mind, such as an unrealistic expectation. Picture chains being on you and Jesus paying to have those chains removed. What would freedom feel and look like?

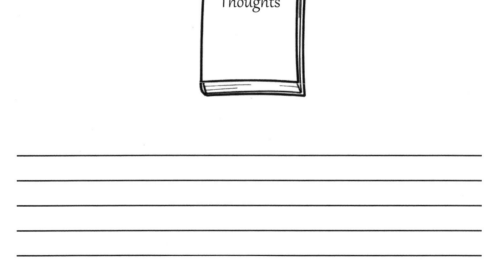

Thoughts

_____

_____

_____

_____

_____

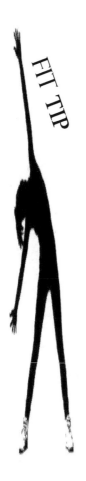

FIT TIP

Mind trip, false grip!

"Dieting" in the sense of restricting yourself from calories can not only be a mind trip, but is also a false grip. In other words, you think you have a handle on the situation but it can actually work against you. It does not always help you shed pounds and you can end up worse off than before. When you stop eating calories, you stop producing the hormone leptin, which is needed to lose weight.

Instead of dieting, the best thing to do is to create a lifestyle change of eating well-balanced, nutritional foods in proper proportion and incorporating some form of exercise. Foods to steer clear of that create a sensitivity to leptin are fried foods with trans-fat, wheat-based foods, which cause internal inflammation, soy in the form of soybean oil and corn, which is genetically modified (as in the ever-prevalent high fructose corn syrup). High fructose corn syrup creates addiction and is linked to the rising rate of obesity, as it is in many foods and drinks and is being added to many that we don't expect, such as wheat bread and baby foods. Read labels carefully.

Day 13

SPLENDOR

"They will be called oaks of righteousness, a planting of the Lord for the display of His splendor."

Isaiah 61:3 (NIV)

"They spread their wings and soar like eagles, they run and don't get tired."

Isaiah 40:32 (MSG)

Food for Thought

The motivation behind getting your body fit is, not as an obligation, but as the joy of being able to use it as an instrument of expression. Your body is a display of splendor for His glory.

Eric Liddell, an Olympic runner, whom the movie *Chariots of Fire* is about, said, "God made me fast. And when I run, I feel His pleasure." You may feel that way when you run or dance. When you do something athletic, your body feels like it can fly when it is in shape. Scientifically, the body releases endorphins when you exercise that actually make you joyful. That's a good motivation to get your body in shape or to train - to get to that point where you feel God's pleasure.

What is something you feel that way about? Fill in the blank: "When I _____, I feel God's pleasure." It could be something athletic or artistic or something as simple as walking or taking a class. What would it take to get to the point where you could feel that? You don't have to be an expert at something to feel God's pleasure doing it. His pleasure can feel like peace, joy or love. Let God show you how to sense His pleasure in the things you do.

Thoughts

_____

_____

_____

_____

_____

_____

_____

_____

_____

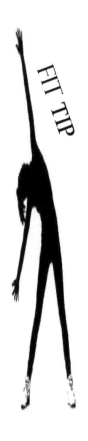

FIT TIP

Runner's high from exercise!

Vigorous **aerobic exercise** can stimulate the release of endorphins in the bloodstream, leading to an effect known as a "runner's high". Laughter may also stimulate endorphin production.

The most effective runner's workout for the average person is intermittent running (sprints) with walking and/or jogging. Running burns about 100 calories per mile for the average person, while walking burns about half of that.

Other ways to fulfill the recommended two hour average of moderate to vigorous-intensity aerobic activity per week are a brisk thirty minute walk four days a week, one hour spin or Zumba class twice a week, or a combination thereof. If you are trying to lose weight, it is recommended that you exercise at least thirty minutes a day, along with eating healthy - and laughing a lot!

TRUST IS HEALTH TO YOUR FLESH

Inspiration

"Trust in the Lord with all your heart,
And lean not on your own understanding;
In all your ways acknowledge Him,
And He shall direct your paths…
It will be health to your flesh,
And strength to your bones."

Proverbs 3:5-6,8 (NKJV)

Food for Thought

When you trust God to help you in every area of your life, He can help direct your path. Acknowledge Him, or let Him in on, everything you do or all your ways. That includes your physical, emotional, relational, and financial concerns. As you trust in Him, not doing it all on your own, He brings health to your flesh and strength to your bones. If you struggle with food, alcohol, sexual, or self-image issues, or whatever it may be concerning your body, try acknowledging Him when you are in the middle of the struggle. Lean on Him instead of trying to combat it yourself. Tell Him what you're thinking, even in the middle of it. He can give you strength and direct your path.

Activate

Is there an area you are not acknowledging God in or letting Him in? Picture it like a house and you only let Him in certain rooms, but keep the door shut on the other rooms so they remain dark. He has the key to light and life, strength and health. Invite Him into that room now. Write what you are exposing to Him and listen to how He feels about it. What is He saying to you? You might be surprised.

Thoughts

_____

_____

_____

_____

_____

_____

_____

_____

_____

_____

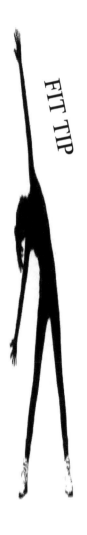

FIT TIP

The core can open every other door!

Just as your mental and physical health are affected by the central GI tract, your body strength centers in the core. The core is located lower than most people think or target while doing sit-ups such as crunches which target the upper abdominals. The core is actually located between the belly button and the pelvis in the crisscross muscles of the transverse abdominals. Pilates focuses on this area.

The heart of exercise is a strong core. In physical training, the core can control, centralize and stabilize everything else. A strong core can accelerate other areas of training. If you do not have a strong core, you are more susceptible to injury.

A good exercise for the core is the Pilates Hundred.

1. Lie on your back with your legs bent in tabletop position (45 degree uprise with your shins and ankles parallel to the floor). Inhale
2. Exhale and press your core down to the floor, scooping out and away as you bring your head up, curling your upper spine up off the floor to the base of your shoulder blades. Keep the shoulders sliding down and engaged in the back as you lengthen into a "C" position (or "C curve").
3. Your arms extend straight and low, just a few inches off the floor, with the fingertips reaching for the far wall.
4. Take five short breaths in and five short breaths out. While doing so, move your arms in a controlled up and down manner - a small but dynamic pumping of the arms. Ten sets of ten (five breaths in and five out) will equal 100 which is why it's called The Hundred.

Day 15

YOUR BODY IS A TEMPLE

"Do you not know that your body is the temple of the Holy Spirit who is in you, whom you have from God."

I Corinthians 6:19 (NKJV)

"Jesus said... 'Destroy this temple, and in three days I will raise it up.' Then the Jews said, 'It has taken forty-six years to build this temple, and will You raise it up in three days?' But He was speaking of the temple of His body."

John 2:19-21 (NKJV)

Food for Thought

In the Old Testament, the temple was where the people would meet God. It was destroyed when the Babylonians took the Jews into exile and took forty-six years to rebuild. In the New Testament, Jesus said you could connect to God through Him - He is the temple. When you have His Spirit within you, you are the temple that houses the heart of God.

If you think about your body being filled with the Spirit of God, you may treat it with more respect. It is just as important to keep it shining on the inside as it is on the outside. Sometimes that calls for a redecorating or renovating, which goes along with renewing the mind - it is a restoring of the temple. Even if you feel it has been destroyed or it's taken forty-six years to become what it is, with Him, you can raise up your body on a daily basis to be the temple that shines His light.

Activate

If you were to redecorate, renovate, or rebuild (raise) your temple (body), what would that look like? Is there an area in your heart that needs restoring? Ask God what the beauty of His temple looks like in you.

Thoughts

_____

_____

_____

_____

_____

_____

_____

_____

_____

_____

_____

_____

_____

_____

_____

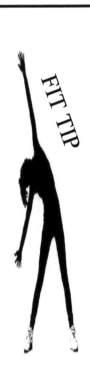

FIT TIP

Restore with more - the Afterburn!

There is a window within ninety minutes post-workout for restoring the body with ultimate carb and protein ingestion and absorption. It is the Afterburn Effect, which can help you burn more calories long after you've left the gym. Another name for it is EPOC (excess post-exercise oxygen consumption). The high-intensity training sessions force the body to work harder to build its oxygen stores back up.

This state where the body's metabolism is elevated following exercise is the best time to replenish and burn calories. Protein and carbs are the most beneficial. Eating protein within thirty minutes after your work-out is a sure muscle metabolism booster!

Day 16

BODILY EXPRESSION

Inspiration

"Offer your bodies as a living sacrifice, holy and pleasing to God—this is your true and proper worship."

Romans 12:1 (NIV)

"Then David danced before the Lord with all his might.. David said, "I will celebrate before the Lord. I will become even more undignified."

2 Samuel 6:14,21-22

"For in Him we live and move and have our being."

Acts 17:28 (NIV)

Food for Thought

David used his body as a full expression of his thanks to God for giving him victory. He was so full of praise and gratitude that he let himself go even to the point of being willing to appear undignified. He put all his might into worship in this way. David was a warrior, a strong and mighty man of valor, yet he allowed himself to be free with his body to express gratitude, even if it meant looking foolish.

What would it look like if you were to let your body go to fully express what is inside with unfiltered praise and gratitude? There is something freeing about physical expression through movement, even if you are not a dancer.

Activate

Let yourself go. Put on music and try what David did - dancing with all your might! Whatever that may look like. Think of something you want to express and create that image or feeling in your body. For instance, if you are expressing gratitude, you might lift your arms up in the air. If you are expressing pain, you might wrap your arms around your waist. Write about your experience or what God showed you through that. If that is difficult, find another way your body can express gratitude or praise fully and freely or just write with all your might!

Thoughts

_____

_____

_____

_____

_____

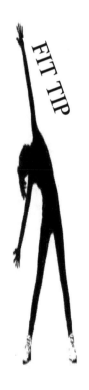

Expression and variety are the spice of life - that includes in foods!

Some seasonings can spice up your meals with flavor, along with the added benefit of curbing appetite and speeding up metabolism, thus having a fat-burning ability. Hot, spicy foods contribute to satiety (the feeling of fullness after eating). In addition to making people feel full faster, chili powder and many other spices have a thermogenic effect. This results in the body heating itself from within, which revs up the metabolism. Some studies have found that adding thermogenic spices to a meal can increase the number of calories burned by 25% for up to an hour after the meal. Not to mention add some zest! The following spices have been shown to have this effect to some degree: Black pepper, chili powder, cayenne pepper, cumin, mustard, turmeric, ginger, and cinnamon. They also carry benefits for the blood and antioxidant qualities.

Day 17

SOURCE OF STRENGTH

"My grace is sufficient for you, for my power is made perfect in weakness. Therefore I will boast all the more gladly about my weaknesses, so that Christ's power may rest on me."

2 Corinthians 12:9 (NIV)

"I can do all this through Him who gives me strength."

Philippians 4:13 (NIV)

Food for Thought

The irony of the Kingdom of God is that when you are weak, He is strong in you. When you are humble, He lifts you up. The first are last and the last, first.

If you are weak in a certain area of your life, it could be a great point of surrender for you. If you give your weakness over to God and surrender it to Him, He can come in and make you strong with the power of His Spirit, which is stronger than what you can do on your own. If you are struggling in an area, such as with food or exercise, let Him come in and give you the strength. In Him you can do all things because His strength has no limits and His grace in those situations is sufficient. It is simply enough to give it to Him and allow Him to release, cover and empower you..

Activate

What is an area you feel weak in or lack self-discipline? Ask God to fill your weakness with His strength. Write what you look like cloaked in the cape of God's strength.

Thoughts

_____

_____

_____

_____

_____

_____

_____

_____

_____

_____

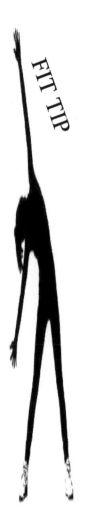

FIT TIP

What's white may not be right!

One irony in foods is that many white foods, which appear pure, can actually be a detriment to your health. They can cause you to have lower energy, leaving you unsatisfied, which increases cravings and causes weight gain.

The main difference between the healthful and unhealthful foods is processing. Refined and processed foods are foods that are altered from their original state usually to create a longer shelf life at the cost of losing nutrients. Processing also strips food of natural fiber. Most white carbs start with flour that has been ground and refined by stripping off the outer layer, where the fiber is located. These refined carbs are less satisfying, making it easy to overeat. Without the fiber to regulate absorption, the body absorbs processed grains and simple sugars relatively quickly. Increased blood sugar triggers a release of insulin, and, in an hour or two after eating, hunger returns.

The most common white foods which have been processed and refined are flour, rice, pasta, bread, crackers, cereal, and simple sugars like table sugar and high-fructose corn syrup.

Of course there are healthier natural, unprocessed white foods, such as onions, cauliflower, turnips, white beans, and white potatoes. These whole foods are some of the right whites!

Day 18

TEMPTATION

"Watch and pray so that you will not fall into temptation. The spirit is willing, but the flesh is weak."

Matthew 26:41 (NIV)

"No temptation has seized you except what is common to man. And God is faithful; He will not let you be tempted beyond what you can bear. But when you are tempted, He will also provide an escape, so that you can stand up under it."

I Corinthians 10:13 (BSB)

Food for Thought

Merriam-Webster defines temptation as "something that causes a strong urge or desire to have or do something and especially something that is bad, wrong, or unwise." It's usually manifested in the physical form and has to do with the body, although it begins in the mind. The first temptation in history had to do with food and the symbolism behind it. Eve ate the fruit from the tree of the knowledge of good and evil, which was the only forbidden thing in the garden. God forbids things that He knows will be harmful to us. It was when evil was recognized by Adam and Eve after they ate the fruit that shame and self-consciousness entered into the human experience.

Satan knows he can make you feel shameful and insecure when you give in to a temptation that will produce bad fruit in your life - whether it's drinking to excess or eating things in portions that are harmful to your body. This affects both your health and self-image.

The best way to fight temptation of any kind is to watch and pray. Be alert to recognize it and call temptation what it is. Then be honest with yourself and God. Talk to Him when you are feeling tempted. This brings what is hidden and shameful into the open. Everyone deals with this in one form or another. Bring it into the light with Him. He is the one who will help you. He does not tempt. Satan is the one who is the tempter. God does not revel in teasing you. He is always there to provide a way of escape into His loving arms. Remember, where you are weak, He is strong.

If it happens over again, continue talking to God in the middle of whatever you are dealing with. His presence will pervade. The warfare always starts with the voice of evil trying to separate us from good (God), so if you feel separated, He said He is always with you. You can stand on that truth.

Activate

What is a temptation you struggle with? Talk to God about it. Ask Him to show you the plan of escape so you can recognize it when it comes and He can give you the strength during those times. What do you see on the other end of the victory over the struggle?

Thoughts

_____

_____

_____

_____

_____

_____

_____

_____

_____

_____

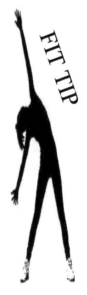

The drink that keeps you afloat!

You need to drink at least half of your body weight in ounces of water a day to keep your body hydrated and functioning at its best. If you weigh 150 lbs. you would drink at least 75 ounces of water a day. It also helps you lose weight if you drink at least eight ounces of water before meal times, as you will tend to eat less. It's recommended to drink at least eight ounces of water when you wake up and eight ounces before you sleep. Note that your body can only absorb four ounces every fifteen minutes, so it's good to spread it out a bit. Drinking the right amount of water daily can actually speed up your metabolic rate and help to curb overeating.

Day 19

FASTING

"So Jesus said to them, ...for assuredly, I say to you, if you have faith as a mustard seed, you will say to this mountain, 'Move from here to there,' and it will move; and nothing will be impossible for you. However, this kind does not go out except by prayer and fasting."

Matthew 17:19-21 (NKJV)

Food for Thought

When you need faith that moves mountains in your life, prayer and fasting work hand-in-hand. Fasting, for spiritual reasons, is basically not eating to focus on prayer. It allows you to take authority in the spiritual realm as you do the opposite of what first separated man from God, in order to connect with Him. Adam and Eve ate something that *wasn't* allowed. When you fast, you voluntarily deny yourself of something that *is* allowed. It is not about rules of not being able to have something, but rather it is about choosing relationship with God over something you can have. Especially if what needs to be broken, the mountain that needs to be moved in your life, has to do with strongholds of food or mindsets about it. It is taking authority over it by simply putting your focus on something higher.

Spiritually, fasting is good to cleanse the soul and create a clearer path to hearing from heaven without distraction and with a disciplined heart to be able to receive all God says. Physically, fasting (or cleansing) can detoxify the body and prepare it to receive the nutritional value that can regenerate and energize you.

Activate

Is there a mountain in your life that needs moving? Name the mountain. What could you fast, or do without, to set your focus on hearing from God and standing in faith? What is on the other side of that mountain? Ask God to show you and to give you the strength to fast - even for a short time. Write what He tells you during that time.

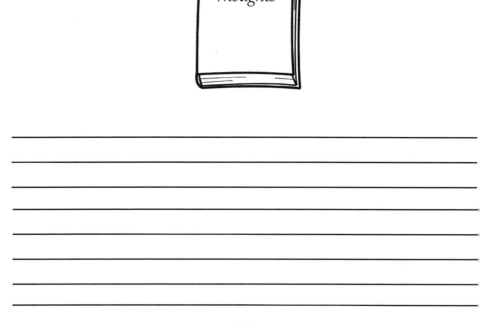

Thoughts

_____

_____

_____

_____

_____

_____

_____

_____

_____

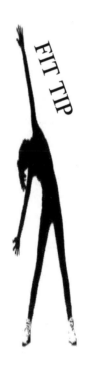

FIT TIP

A "fast" that doesn't "slow" you down!

When you fast with just water, your body goes into a state of ketosis or starvation mode. It makes it hard to burn fat and your body actually starts eating away at muscle. The most effective way to do it long- or short-term is to have protein days along with intermittent high nutritional fasting days, where your metabolism continues working. This also helps to cleanse the gut in a beneficial way, ridding unhealthy bacteria while maintaining the good bacteria. When you fast in this way, it helps cleanse your mind and spirit while cleansing your body in a healthy and attainable way.

A link to a recommended cleanse program with nutritional fasting days can be found in the back of the book. (3)

Day 20

PHYSICAL TRAINING

Inspiration

"Physical training is good, but training for Godliness is much better, promising benefits in this life, and in the life to come."

1 Timothy 4:8 (NLT)

"Do you not know that in a race all the runners run, but only one gets the prize? Run in such a way as to get the prize. Everyone who competes in the games goes into strict training. They do it to get a crown that will not last, but we do it to get a crown that will last forever."

1 Corinthians 9:24-25 (NIV)

Food for Thought

You exercise so that you can be healthy and feel fit to do all God has called you to do, but you have to also keep it in perspective. Physical training has to go along with spiritual training. Don't negate one for the other. Take God with you and include Him.

When you are disciplined in spirit and soul, it is for an eternal glory. Physical training is good, but temporary. God loves that you are taking care of the vessel and instrument of your body as long as you are not under the law of it or obsessed to the point of excluding Him.

Activate

Walk and talk! Walking is a great way to communicate with God and be physically training at the same time. Try going for a walk and using your phone to record your thoughts as you walk. Speak what He is saying to you. When you get back you can write what you heard and spoke into the recorder.

Thoughts

_____

_____

_____

_____

_____

_____

_____

_____

_____

_____

_____

_____

_____
_____
_____
_____
_____
_____
_____
_____
_____
_____
_____
_____
_____

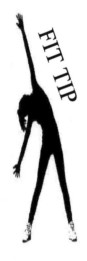

Walk + Water + Word = Win

The three positive "W's" to live by are Walk, Water and Word. They are the easiest way to a winning life of health. If nothing else, remember these three "W's daily.

Walking (twenty minutes a day), drinking the recommended amount of Water (half your bodyweight), and reading the Word, can keep you refreshed and on the right path to Wholeness.

Part Three

SOUL

SOUL

The soul is the incorporeal (without a human body) and immortal essence of a living being. It is the immaterial part of a human body - the emotional part of human nature that seats feelings or sentiments. Many associate it with the core of the body which is basically the gut. When people speak of "gut reaction" they are referring to intuitive - emotional response. The Greek word for "soul" is *psykhe* and is where we get the word psyche: affections, will, desire, emotions, mind, reason and understanding. It is the inner self or the essence of life.

The Bible associates soul with living being, person, desire, appetite, emotion and passion. It is your inner being or that which breaths.

> *"He has put Him to grief when you make His soul an offering for sin,....He shall see the labor of His soul, and be satisfied... For He shall bear their iniquities."*
> *Isaiah 53:10, 11(NKJV)*

When you understand that the cross was not just about the physical pain but the bearing of your soul griefs, it helps put into light the fullness of the sacrifice for your well-being. Jesus understands the depth of your heart and emotions as He felt every hurt or emptiness you would ever feel all at one time.

In order to be healthy in the soul, you often need healing in your emotions. This can include needing to dissipate fear, guilt, despair and regret. Often you have to release offense, actively choose to forgive and break unhealthy emotional ties (soul ties).

Sentiment can keep you locked or paralyzed in the past, but when you let go of the disappointment or disillusionment, you can move forward to restore your soul to be free and allow healthy emotions in so your soul will prosper and you can pursue the desires and passions that lead to wholeness and life.

117

SOUL

The soul is your center
Acknowledged as the core
The immaterial essence
Of emotions you store.
Kindness and sympathy
The deeply felt moral part
That helps you appreciate
Splendor in beauty and art.
Regret, guilt and perfection
Can paralyze your soul.
Keeping you locked in fear
Far away from being whole.
Focusing on your failures,
Disappointment or despair
Leaves your soul longing
For grace, hope, and care.
Holding on to old offense
Can toxically take its toll
The healing of forgiveness
Brings freedom to the soul.

Savory soul-seasoning
Healing hearts broken
Like a sweet honeycomb
Are pleasant words spoken.
The healing of the soul
Goes beyond the core
The letting go of your life
Brings life forevermore.
Jesus has compassion
For every emotional pain
He became a soul offering
Bearing all hurt and shame.
He binds your broken heart
He wants to set you free
Releasing soul wounds
For all you're created to be.
You have true life and peace
As you receive His love for you
Your soul is fit for freedom
To love yourself and others, too.

Day 21

FORGIVE YOURSELF

Inspiration

"Jesus replied, 'Love the Lord your God with all your heart and with all your soul and with all your mind. This is the greatest commandment. And the second is like it. 'Love your neighbor as yourself'"

Matthew 22:37-39 (NIV)

"Then Peter came to Jesus and asked, 'Lord, how many times shall I forgive my brother or sister who sins against me? Up to seven times?' Jesus answered, 'I tell you, not seven times, but seventy-seven times."

Matthew 18:21, 22 (NIV)

"If we tell Him our sins, He is faithful and we can depend on Him to forgive us our sins. He will make our lives clean."

I John 1:9 (NLT)

Food for Thought

One of the biggest things that keeps your soul from being free is unforgiveness. Jesus said to forgive your brother or sister seventy times seven. In order to be able to do that, you have to forgive yourself since the second greatest commandment is to love your neighbor as yourself. Loving yourself includes forgiving yourself, which releases you to forgive others as well.

You may be holding yourself in bondage through something you have not forgiven yourself for. The first step is understanding that God has already forgiven you. All He wants you to do is tell Him (confess) and He is faithful to forgive. Then you have to release yourself from it. Forgive yourself - even if it happens again or it takes seventy times seven times - you have to continue to forgive yourself and walk in grace. Give yourself the grace God has already given you.

Activate

Ask God if there is anything you still hold yourself responsible for from your past that you need to forgive yourself for. Is there anything that you are dealing with in the present that you need to forgive yourself for? Even if you feel you have failed over and over in this area. It may be as simple as failing to stick to a nutrition or exercise plan. Or perhaps you stumbled in what you would consider a big way. Release it to God and free yourself from self-condemnation. Write a declaration: I forgive you,____ (your name), for _____.

Thoughts

_____

_____

_____

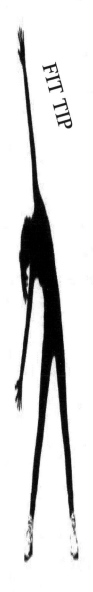

FIT TIP

Forgive and live!

Unforgiveness is classified in medical books as a disease. Dr. Steven Standiford, chief of surgery at the Cancer Treatment Centers of America, says refusing to forgive makes people sick and keeps them that way. Harboring these negative emotions, along with anger and hate, creates a state of chronic anxiety which produces excess adrenaline and cortisol, depleting the production of natural killer cells that help fight cancer.

Anger also suppresses the immune system. It causes stress, which decreases IgA (immunoglobulin A), the protective coating for the cells against invading bacteria and viruses. This leaves you more vulnerable to respiratory problems such as colds or flu.

One minute of anger weakens the immune system for four to five hours, while one minute of laughter boosts the immune system for twenty-four hours by decreasing stress hormones. Laughter also relaxes your body for up to forty-five minutes, releases endorphins, protects the heart by increasing blood flow, and burns calories. One study showed that laughing for ten to fifteen minutes a day can burn about forty calories - enough to lose three or four pounds over the course of a year. A study in Norway also found that people with a strong sense of humor outlived those who don't laugh as much. The difference was particularly notable for those battling cancer.

Laugh yourself to health!

"A joyful heart is good medicine"

Proverbs 17:22 (NASB)

FORGIVE OTHERS

Inspiration

"You must be kind to each other. Think of the other person. Forgive other people just as God forgave you..."

Ephesians 4:32 (NLV)

"Then the master of that servant was moved with compassion, released him, and forgave him the debt.... '

"...Then his master, after he had called him, said to him, 'You wicked servant! I forgave you all that debt because you begged me. Should you not also have had compassion on your fellow servant, just as I had pity on you?'"

Matthew 18:27, 33 (NKJV)

Food for Thought

These verses from Matthew are from a parable Jesus told concerning forgiveness. It is about a servant who begs a king for patience to pay off his debt so he and his family would not be sold. The king has compassion on the servant and releases him and forgives his big debt. The servant turns around and demands a fellow servant to pay a small debt he owed him. When the fellow servant begs for patience to pay off the debt, he has him thrown into prison. When the king finds out, he is angry that the servant did not show the same compassion that he showed him. He has him thrown in prison to be tortured until he can pay all that is owed him.

Because God has forgiven all of your debt (sins), He wants you to have the same compassion and forgiveness for those who have sinned against you. It is releasing them of the debt you feel they owe you. It frees your soul.

You may have heard the saying that when you hold bitterness or offense in your heart, it is like drinking poison and expecting the other person to die. It hurts you more than the other person and holds your soul in bondage. So, even if they do not ask for forgiveness or show signs of being sorry, by releasing forgiveness it frees the space in your own heart that was being taken up by offense to be open to love. When you forgive you are not agreeing with what someone else did to you, you are just releasing them from the debt you feel they owe you from it. God will pay you back with His Kingdom mercy and grace and fill that space in your soul with His unconditional love and peace that passes understanding. You'll know you are free when you are able to pray blessings on that person.

Activate

Ask God to show you someone who may have hurt you or sinned against you. It may be someone who has caused you hurt or contributed to an unhealthy self-image or destructive habits that have been hard to break. What do you feel they owe you? Ask God to help you release them of their debt. Bless them. Ask Him to show you how He will fill that space in your soul with His love and grace to free you.

Thoughts

_____
_____
_____
_____
_____
_____
_____
_____
_____
_____
_____
_____
_____
_____
_____
_____
_____
_____
_____

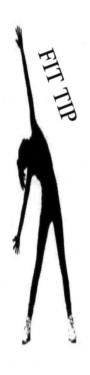

FIT TIP

Poison (toxin) control!

Just as unforgiveness is toxic to your soul, there are toxins (poisonous substances) that enter your body through what you eat, drink, breathe or what contacts your skin. **T**oxicity is one of the biggest hindrances to health, along with **D**eficiency, **O**verweight and **S**tress. Peter Greenlaw* addresses these in his book <u>The TDOS Syndrome</u> ®. The first step is to recognize these contributing factors, known as TDOS, and then take steps to support your body in naturally detoxifying through nutrition, exercise and nutritional fasting (or cleansing). (3)

More information on this can be found at <u>www.SusanSilvestri.com</u>.

Day 23

HOPE DURING TIMES OF DISAPPOINTMENT OR DESPAIR

Inspiration

"The Spirit of the Lord God is upon Me, because the Lord has anointed Me to preach good tidings to the poor; He has sent me to bind up the brokenhearted, to proclaim freedom for the captives and release from darkness for the prisoners, ...to comfort all who mourn, ...to bestow on them a crown of beauty instead of ashes, the oil of joy instead of mourning and a garment of praise instead of a spirit of despair."

Isaiah 61:1-3 (NKJV)

Food for Thought

Often, what keeps your soul in darkness is despair or disappointment, either in circumstances of life or in yourself. These verses describe the ministry of God's anointed as a healer and messenger of freedom and comfort. Jesus quoted this prophetic word years later, proclaiming that *He* brings good news to the poor, which includes the poor in spirit. *He* heals the broken hearted, which includes disillusionment or disappointment. *He* brings freedom to those in captivity, which includes captive to negative thoughts or patterns. *He* releases prisoners from darkness, which includes the darkness of despair or circumstances. *He* brings beauty from ashes. *He* gives joy for sadness.

When you are feeling depleted or deprived, when you have a broken heart from a relationship or situation, when you feel trapped or imprisoned, when you are despondent, He can comfort your soul and make something beautiful of what seems like ashes. The power of praise casts off oppressive works of darkness and brings light and joy.

When *He* lives in you, you too can carry that message of joy, freedom and hope to others.

Activate

Is there a circumstance that has kept you in darkness or despair? Have you been disappointed in your life about something or disappointed in yourself for some reason? Write it and then release it. You may even write it on a separate piece of paper and burn it. Let God show you how He can bring beauty from the ashes. Ask Him to release you from the prison of those emotions and bring light to your darkness. Ask Him to show you the hope beyond the circumstance.

Thoughts

_____

_____

_____

_____

_____

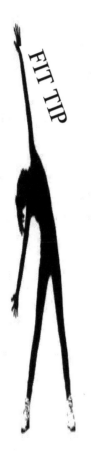

FIT TIP

Bring back your lack!

Just as when your soul is deficient you lose hope, when you are deficient in an area of life, your quality of life potential is inhibited. The deficiency in food sources these days causes a hindrance to health. The second letter "D" in The TDOS Syndrome stands for "Deficiency". Because of pesticides and the lack of nutrients in our soils, even organic food lacks the nutritional trace minerals, digestive enzymes, quality proteins, vitamins, and healthy fats your body needs to thrive. You need 70 minerals every day. Even with the best organic food you get a mere ten minerals (12 % of what you need). According to a UCLA study, it would take forty bags of spinach at one sitting to equal the nutritional level from one bowl of spinach in 1953. It's no longer enough to get everything you need from just food. You need good, absorbable supplements.

There are recommendations for quality nutritional supplements listed in the back of the book. (4)

Day 24

RESTORE THE SOUL

"The Lord is my shepherd;
I shall not want.
He makes me to lie down in green pastures;
He leads me beside the still waters.
He restores my soul."

Psalm 23:1-3 (NKJV)

"If a man owns a hundred sheep, and one of them wanders away, will he
not leave the ninety-nine on the hills and go for the one that wandered
off?"

Matthew 18:12 (NIV)

Food for Thought

God restores your soul in the areas you feel have been compromised, hurt or destroyed. To restore is to bring back or go back to a point of departure. It is the point where you feel it was damaged or you departed from the fullness God intended for you or the vision He gave you.

Even if your loss was due to your own mistake or sin, God is a God of grace and new beginnings. After the Israelites lost their land due to their own rebellion, He promised to restore the land and all that was lost to them. "So I will restore to you the years that the swarming locust has eaten." Joel 2:25 (NKJV)

He restores your soul to the place of peace in green pastures and still waters. He is a loving shepherd who would leave the ninety-nine sheep to come after or restore the one.

Activate

Is there an area in your life where you feel a loss or you feel you departed from God's fullness and need restoring? Sometimes it is on a daily basis that you need to allow God to restore your soul, even if the restoration is needed because of something of your own doing.

If the Lord, your Shepherd were to pick you up and carry you back to a place of green pastures and still waters, what would He be restoring in your life? What is He saying to you in that place of peace?

Thoughts

The loss that restores!

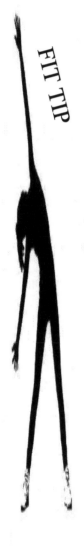

One area of loss that may actually restore your body is weight loss, when done in a healthy manner.

Overweight is the "O" of the TDOS Syndrome. According to the CDC (Centers for Disease Control and Prevention) 70.7% of American adults over twenty are overweight, including 37.9% who are considered obese. The global rate is also on the rise.

One of the biggest factors in overweight is obesogens, the scientific name for toxins stored in your fat cells. These are chemicals we're exposed to every day, which alter the regulatory system that controls your weight—increasing the fat cells you have, decreasing the calories you burn, and even altering the way your body manages hunger.

Obesogens are found everywhere, from high fructose corn syrup to places you wouldn't suspect, such as in Perfluorooctanoic acid (PFOA) found in non-stick, Teflon pans and microwave popcorn bags. Bisphenol-A (BPA) is found in plastic bottles and Phthalates, which are chemicals found in vinyl products, such as air fresheners.

When you support the body's natural detoxification capability with nutritional fasting, you are eliminating many of these toxins from being stored in your fat cells. Giving up soda, with high fructose corn syrup, can play a huge role in ridding your body of obesogens and helping you to lose weight.

OVERCOMING FEAR/PERFECTIONISM

Inspiration

"There is no fear in love. But perfect love drives out fear, because fear has to do with punishment. The one who fears is not made perfect in love."

John 4:18 (NIV)

"Fear of man will prove to be a snare, but whoever trusts in the Lord is kept safe"

Proverbs 29:25 (NIV)

Food for Thought

When your soul is in fear, you stay locked up in your own torment. There are many forms of fear, but a couple of the ones that keep you from being whole are *fear of man* and *fear of failure*.

"Fear of man" means to be more concerned about what people think of you than what God thinks about you or even what you think about yourself. Fear will cause you to have a tendency to compare yourself to others, especially in a world of Facebook and Instagram, which often results in feeling rejection. Since perfect love drives out that fear, when you spend time reflecting on God's love for you and spending time with the One who IS Love itself, you become more confident in who you are and put less weight on what others think of or expect from you.

When you fear failure, you strive for significance through what you do instead of who you are. You are always looking to achieve that big accomplishment instead of appreciating the little steps and relationships, including with yourself, along the way.

Ironically, you may experience perfectionism (expecting yourself to be perfect) out of both fear of man and fear of failure, when in reality, the only thing that can conquer that is "perfect love". Perfect love is God's agape, unconditional love. He is the lover of your soul.

Release the burden of expecting yourself to be perfect and punishing yourself when you do not meet up to your own expectation or what you think others expect of you. If you punish yourself for blowing it when you are attempting to eat healthy and exercise, give yourself grace and trust God to be your strength step-by-step. Don't sit in bondage as you fear your failure, but release it to God and He can free you. Rest in His perfect love for you.

Activate

What is it that you fear? Is there a person or persons whose opinion(s) you are holding in higher value than that of yourself or God? Write the name(s). Write your fears of what they might think. Ask God why that is important to you. Ask Him what His opinion is.

Thoughts

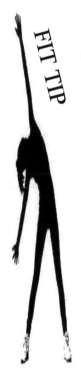

Nutritional best will relieve stress!

Fear can create stress. Stress is the fourth letter of the TDOS Syndrome. According to Stanford Medical School, chronic stress is the #1 killer. It produces high levels of cortisol (the stress hormone), causing insulin spikes which, in turn, cause the body to store fat. It also increases free radicals, which accelerate aging in the body and can be linked to cancer. The three biggest causes of stress are physical, relational, and financial. Staying connected to God, self and others can help. Hopefully this book will inspire that.

Maintaining a good balance of exercise and nutritional supplements can also help lower stress.

There is a good stress-relieving drink containing a blend of plant-based Adaptogens (herbal stress reducers) recommended in the back of the book. (5)

Day 26

FILLING AN EMPTY SOUL

Inspiration

"For He fills the thirsty soul. And He fills the hungry soul with good things."

Psalm 107:9 (NLV)

"No longer will they call you Deserted, or name your land Desolate. But you will be called Hephzibah (my delight is in her) and your land Beulah (married); for the Lord will take delight in you, and your land will be married."

Isaiah 62:4 (NIV)

"Take delight in the Lord, and he will give you the desires of your heart."

Psalm 37:4 (NIV).

"For everyone who asks receives; the one who seeks finds; and to the one who knocks, the door will be opened. Which of you, if your son asks for bread, will give him a stone?"

Matthew 7:8, 9 (NIV)

Food for Thought

Is there an area in your soul you feel is desolate or empty? Maybe you try filling it with food or other things. God says that He will fill those places and that He takes delight in you. When you delight in Him as well, He says He will give you the desires of your heart.

He knows the deepest longings of your soul. When you are feeling forsaken or empty, start by recognizing it, then acknowledge it and trust that God will fill it.

If you are lonely (especially if you are single) or have a longing in your heart that leaves you with an empty pit and makes your soul hungry and thirsty for something missing, don't try filling it with other things. Bring it to God and let Him fill you. Tell Him about the longing in your heart. He *wants* to give you your heart's desire. He does not give His children, you, a stone when you ask for bread. He wants to fill your hunger and emptiness because He loves you.

Activate

What is it that may cause you to overeat or overindulge in other things? Is there something missing that you are trying to fill? Write what you are feeling during those times. Is there a longing in your heart that makes you feel empty? What is missing? Ask God to show you. Maybe it's a desire or dream not yet fulfilled. He wants to fill the desires of your heart.

Thoughts

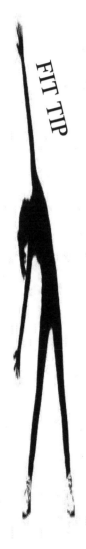

FIT TIP

Quench a thirsty soul with good things, quench a thirsty body with good water!

Many people drink tap or bottled water. However, it was found out that tap water is a "soup" of viruses and bacteria, run-off from farming, including herbicides, pesticides, antibiotics, hormones, pharmaceutical drugs, heavy metals from degrading plumbing...and human and animal wastes, including body fluids from embalming!

We also drink bottled water, but what we don't know is that 25% of bottled water is simply untreated tap water and 75% of bottled water is more acidic than regular tap water. The scary part is that water stored in plastic bottles leaches petro-chemicals called phthalates from the plastic, which has shown to contribute to certain breast cancers in women and erectile dysfunction in men.

Change your water...change your life. The best water to drink is Electrolyzed Reduced Water (ERW), or hydrogen water, which supplies the body with extra free electrons that can be used to help neutralize disease-causing free radicals. This water will help you lose weight, stay younger-looking, have more energy, sleep better, balance your blood sugar, lower blood pressure and cholesterol, lubricate joints, and help with many other health issues. It has forty times the anti-oxidant property of green tea. It is absorbed six times faster than regular water. It is alkalized—and cancer cells cannot grow in an alkaline environment. It has electrolytes (calcium, magnesium, potassium and sodium) that energize and activate your neurons and muscles. This water is what the Japanese call the Fountain of Youth.

You can get this PH balanced alkaline water through a water system. A good one is Kangen Water. (6)

Day 27

GETTING RID OF GUILT

Inspiration

"When I kept silent, my bones wasted away through my groaning all day long. For day and night your hand was heavy on me; My strength was sapped as in the heat of summer. Then I acknowledged my sin to you and did not cover up my iniquity. I said, 'I will confess my transgressions to the Lord.' And you forgave the guilt of my sin."

Psalm 32:3-5 (NIV)

"As far as the east is from the west, so far has he removed our transgressions from us".

Psalm 103:12 (NIV)

"Blessed are those whose iniquities are forgiven, whose sins are covered."

Romans 4:7 (BSB)

Food for Thought

It is not so much your sin as it is the *guilt* of your sin that keeps your soul in bondage. You have been forgiven for your sins as far as the east is from the west. Yet you can hold yourself in bondage and keep your soul from flourishing when you don't hand it to God, trusting Him to remove the guilt by believing fully that He covered it.

Guilt is the opposite of resting in the grace of God and His redemptive work on the cross. When you hold on in your hearts to the guilt, you have not trusted that God meant what He said that your sins are as far as the east is from the west. In other words, He doesn't even remember them.

Hidden sins and the guilt carried along with them not only affects your body, but your soul. Guilt is associated with shame. Shame causes inner torment or sickness of the soul.

Shame can be a core effect of addiction. If you do suffer from any form of addiction, you may need outside help. But the first step is always to acknowledge it. Do not cover it up. Confess to the Lord anything that is hidden. He sees it anyway and knows what is going on. His desire is always communication and relationship with you. Let Him take the burden of the guilt and shame.

Activate

Ask God if there is any hidden area of guilt in your life, heart, or soul. Write what He shows you. Release it to Him. Ask Him to forgive the guilt and remove the shame. Let Him speak to your heart. If there isn't anything, just thank Him that you are free in your soul!

Thoughts

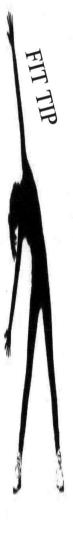

Come clean with food!

The clean eating trend is growing. One of the main foundations of clean eating is cutting out and avoiding processed foods. Doing so will prevent the consumption of unhealthy and sometimes very harmful additives. Processed foods are hard on your body and have been connected to serious health complications, including cardiovascular disease and obesity. They can contain so many bad ingredients that are hard on your liver and difficult for you to digest, and those harmful ingredients and additives are often then stored in the body.

The term "processed food" applies to any food that has been altered from its natural state in some way, either for safety reasons or convenience. Processed foods have been engineered to be "hyper-rewarding," so they trick your brain into eating more than you need, even leading to addiction in some people.

They are also low in fiber, protein and micronutrients, which means they are empty calories. Processed foods are high in unhealthy ingredients like added sugar and refined grains. Try to eat foods that have not been processed.

Remember the One Ingredient Rule. Try eating foods that have just one ingredient, like vegetables and fruits.

Day 28

RELEASE REGRET

"...But Lot's wife looked back, and she became a pillar of salt".

Genesis 19:26 (NIV)

"Brothers and sisters, I do not consider myself yet to have taken hold of it. But one thing I do: Forgetting what is behind and straining toward what is ahead, I press on toward the goal to win the prize for which God has called me heavenward in Christ Jesus."

Philippians 3:13-14 (NIV)

"Because of the Lord's great love we are not consumed, for his compassions never fail. They are new every morning; great is your faithfulness."

Lamentations 3:22-23 (NIV)

Food for Thought

When you live in a place of regret, you paralyze yourself. In Lot's wife's case, she literally became a pillar of salt, but you can figuratively become frozen when you continue to look back in regret or don't let go of what was in the past. The cities were overthrown and there were to be great things ahead, but Lot's wife looked back and mourned the loss of what was. When you let go and move forward, you free yourself to the destiny and fullness God has for you – the prize that is before you. If a runner continues looking back, he will lose momentum for crossing the finish line. Keep your eyes on the prize, knowing that God's mercies are new every morning, so even something you may regret can turn into something victorious.

Even in the areas of nutrition and fitness, you should not be paralyzed by regret if you fail to stick to your expectation. Don't stay stuck in self-sabotage. Instead, take each new day as it comes, letting go of any unfulfilled expectations and keep looking forward to the prize God has ahead. His desire is for you to walk in freedom and fullness and not be stifled or frozen in regret.

Activate

Is there a regret that keeps you paralyzed or looking back? What is the prize ahead that God wants you to focus on?

Thoughts

_____

_____

_____

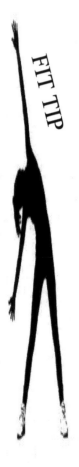

Salt of the earth!

Salt is the most common seasoning mentioned in the Bible. Salt was a vital mineral that was not only essential to life, but also preserved other foods critical for survival. Salt was so important that it was also often used as a form of currency or as a unit of exchange.

Although salt is essential for the body, you need to watch sodium intake. The average daily sodium intake for Americans is 3,400 milligrams, an excessive amount that raises blood pressure and poses health risks. In general, Americans should limit daily sodium consumption to 2,300 milligrams. That is the RDA for salt equivalent to 2.3 grams or 1 tsp.

Sodium is necessary for the body to function. It binds water and maintains intracellular and extracellular fluids in the right balance. That is why top athletes will take salt tablets so that they don't get dehydrated by sweating all the fluids out. That, along with potassium, calcium and magnesium, can also help keep your muscles from cramping.

FIT TIP

Day 29

SWEETS FOR THE SOUL

Inspiration

"Pleasant words are like a honeycomb; sweetness to the soul and health to the bones."

Proverbs 16:24 (NKJV)

"Anxiety in the heart of man causes depression, but a good word makes it glad."

Proverbs 16:24 (NKJV)

"Death and life are in the power of the tongue, and those who eat it will eat its fruit."

Proverbs 18:21

"Speaking to one another with psalms, hymns, and songs from the Spirit, sing and make music from your heart to the Lord."

Ephesians 5:19 (NIV)

"Lay up these words of mine in your heart and in your soul...speaking of them when you sit in your house, when you walk by the way, when you lie down, and when you rise up...write them on the doorposts of your house and on your gates."

Deuteronomy 11:18-20 (NIV)

Food for Thought

The words you hear and speak can really hurt your heart and soul and can even affect your physical health. The old saying, "sticks and stones may break my bones, but names will never hurt me" does not apply – at least not to your soul. Negative words can damage your self-image, confidence and identity. Positive words can lift you up and create an atmosphere for your soul to be fed and prosper.

The first three verses in the Inspiration section, about the impact of words, come from Solomon, who is considered to be the wisest man who ever lived.

If there were negative words spoken over you in your life, you do not need to be defined by them. It is never too late to speak over yourself the truth of how God sees you. Sometimes, the same negative words spoken over you can be turned around to be the very thing that makes you exceptional. For instance, if you were called a "crybaby" when you were a child, you may have a gift of sensitivity and compassion.

Break off any words spoken over you or that you have spoken over yourself, such as, "I'm fat" or "I'm ugly". Even words such as "diet" or "calories" can carry negative, burdensome connotations. Replace these words with "nourishment" or "energy". Food is not your enemy – it is a friend. Used the proper way, it is sweetness to the soul and health to your bones.

When you are discouraged or in a state of depression, try speaking out loud, or singing, words or verses that are true that you may not necessarily feel. *I am a loved child of the King. Your promises are true. You do see my heart and you will meet my every need.* Speak to one another the same way.

God told the Israelites in Deuteronomy to speak about His promises and words of truth all the time, night and day. He said to write them on their doorposts. This was to remind them of all He had done, who He was and who they were to Him. Try posting His promises and words of truth on your refrigerator and around your home to lay them up in your heart and soul. Speak them out loud.

Speak life!

Activate

f you have had any negative words spoken over you that have affected your life, write them down. Next to that, write a counter or opposite word, such as the one in the example - "crybaby" and "compassionate". Maybe someone called you "fat" or "ugly". The truth would be that you are "perfectly proportioned" and "a crown of beauty". Cross out the negative and keep the positive. Ask God what words He would speak over you or speak into existence for our life. It could even be the meaning of your name.

Thoughts

_____

_____

_____

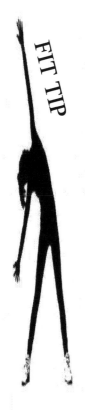

There's nothing sweet about sugary drinks!

Americans drink about 22% of their total calories, much of which is sweetened with sugar or high fructose corn syrup. Sugary drinks are the most fattening things you can put into your body because liquid sugar calories don't get registered by the brain in the same way as calories from solid foods, so when you drink them, you end up consuming more calories.

One can of soda has, an average, 40 grams of sugar (about ten sugar packets). The RDA for sugar is 25 milligrams (about six teaspoons) which is .025 grams. All 150 calories of the soda come from sugar. If you drink one can per day, you are drinking 54,750 extra calories per year, which adds roughly fifteen pounds. This is a large contributor to obesity and type 2 diabetes. Although sodas are probably the worst, keep in mind that fruit juices also have high sugar content.

Sugar also feeds candida, which is a genus of yeasts found in gut flora that can lead to Leaky Gut Syndrome and bloated bellies, which ultimately affects your mind and mood.

There's nothing sweet about that!

Day 30

PEACE IN YOUR SOUL

Inspiration

"Do not be anxious about anything, but in every situation, by prayer and petition, with thanksgiving, present your requests to God. And the peace of God, which transcends all understanding, will guard your hearts and your minds in Christ Jesus."

Philippians 4:6-7 (NIV)

"And we know that in all things God works for the good of those who love Him, who have been called according to His purpose."

Romans 8:28 (NIV)

"Therefore I tell you, do not worry about your life, what you will eat or drink..."

Matthew 6:25 (NIV)

Food for Thought

Anxiety and worry keep your soul from being at peace. This is true even when you worry about what you will eat or drink. The remedy is to go against your natural inclination to strive, to fix, or dwell on your situation. Instead, pray, present your circumstance and request to God, and give Him thanks. That is why it is good to give thanks at meals as a reminder. He feeds you with good things.

159

He holds the answers to all your worries and has already gone before you to cause all things to work together for your good, no matter how bad they may seem.

The famous hymn, *"It is Well with My Soul"*, was written by Horatio G. Spafford in 1873. Horatio wrote it after experiencing a devastating circumstance in his life. He had sent his family ahead on a ship to England. He had business to attend to and was to take a later ship to meet them. The ship his family was on tragically sank when it collided with an iron sailing vessel, killing his four daughters. His wife barely survived and he was on his way to meet her. As he passed over the place the ship had gone down, he could not sleep and said to himself, "It is well; the will of God be done." In the midst of his devastating circumstance, he found a supernatural "peace that passes understanding" (Philippians 4:7) that only God can give. He later wrote the song about that moment.

God will guard your heart from being restless and your mind from dwelling on the negative when you focus on Him and what is true, right and praiseworthy. When you stay in a space of gratitude and trust, the problem becomes smaller and the solution bigger. The burden becomes lighter as you lay it at His feet in petition and prayer.

When you petition, you are making a request to a person in authority or power, asking for some favor, mercy, or other benefit. Only His supernatural power can bring the peace that passes understanding to your circumstance. He calms your heart and mind and puts a guard around it to protect your soul.

Activate

Write your request, petition, and/or prayer to God. If there is anything worrying you, release it. Write out nutrition and fitness goals that don't make you anxious, but energize you toward feeling good. Ask God how to direct your choices and guard your heart.

Thoughts

_____
_____
_____
_____
_____
_____
_____
_____
_____
_____
_____
_____
_____
_____
_____
_____
_____
_____
_____
_____

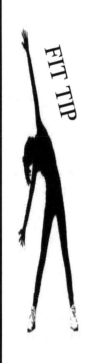

FIT TIP

Find peace through sleep!

When you sleep, you find peace of heart and peace of mind. According to the Mayo Clinic, adults require 7-9 hours of sleep. Lack of sleep contributes to depression and stress. In order to sleep better, try not to eat 2-3 hours before going to sleep to keep your digestive system from having to work overtime. Also try keeping your later meal lighter with a heartier breakfast and lunch meal. Alcohol is not conducive to good sleep. If you do struggle with sleep, there is a good natural sleep support supplement with melatonin listed in the back of the book. (7)

The average person weighing 150 pounds actually burns 95 calories an hour sleeping and someone weighing 115 pounds will burn 45 calories.

Part Four

SPIRIT

SPIRIT

The Spirit is the force within a person that is believed to give the body life, energy, and power; the inner quality or nature of a person (Merriam Webster.) It is the vital principle in humans, mediating between body and soul.

The Latin word is *spiritus,* meaning breath, and in Hebrew, it is *Ruach,* meaning *Breath of Life.* In Greek, it is *pneuma,* meaning the capacity to respond to God. When you respond to Him and allow His Spirit to breathe life into you and empower, comfort, anoint (bless), counsel, and guide you, your spirit is made healthy and whole.

God *spoke* all other creation into being, but with humans, He *breathed* His Spirit into them. It is this intimate act of breathing His own Spirit into you that sets you apart.

A healthy spirit is fed by listening to God's voice, as you have been doing through listening and journaling what He is speaking to your heart. You can recognize when His Spirit is speaking to you because it looks and feels like love, which is the fruit of the Spirit. When you understand His enormous, unconditional love for you, you are freer to hear His true voice.

When you are led by the Spirit, you are empowered to live the life you are meant to, the one God breathed into you. It's not by might or power, but by His Spirit that you can have the discipline and strength to become fit and fully all you are intended to be.

SPIRIT

The spirit can be willing
But the flesh can be weak
Stay connected to the vine
As God's kingdom you seek.
Put on His full armor daily
Take up His shield and sword
"Not by might, nor by power
By My Spirit," says the Lord.
He will give you victory
That comes from on high
Not just to walk and run
But to have wings to fly.
He came not to condemn
He came to set you free
To the abundance of life
For which He holds the key.
As you wholly love the Lord
With heart, mind, spirit, soul
He'll keep you kingdom fit
He will make you whole.
He'll give you eyes to see
A mind focused on truth
A rejoicing soul set free
A body renewed as youth.

He'll restore years stolen
Your empty heart he'll fill.
Soaring on eagles wings
He'll take you higher still.
He'll soak you with wisdom
He'll strengthen your root
He'll water you with love
So you produce good fruit.
He won't leave you behind
An orphan spirit he'll unmask
He'll give exceedingly more
Than you could dream or ask.
He'll give you revelations
He'll guide your every day
He'll set your feet to walk in
The light, the truth, the way.
His heart is ever for you
He died so you could see
The fullness of His love
That truly sets your spirit free.

Day 31

SOURCE OF THE SPIRIT

Inspiration

"I am the vine, you are the branches. If you remain in me and I in you, you will bear much fruit; apart from me you can do nothing."

John 15:5 (NIV)

"Trust in the Lord with ALL your heart and lean not on your understanding; In ALL your ways acknowledge Him, and He shall direct your paths."

Proverbs 3:5 (NKJV)

Food for Thought

As you stay connected to the source of nourishment which is God's love, through reading His words and spending time with Him in conversation, which entails speaking *and* listening, He will direct you toward what will bring about the vision He has given you for your life, which will produce fruit.

God invites you to acknowledge Him in ALL your ways. This includes anything you feel you are struggling with. No matter what the situation, you are free to bring Him into it. Let Him be involved and He will direct you and help put you on the right path. When you are doing things through the nourishment or strength of

169

being connected to His vine, it is not a struggle to produce fruit - it comes naturally out of the outflow of the life source of the Holy Spirit.

Activate

Is there any area of your life you feel like you have to tackle alone or where you are striving in your own power to be productive? Maybe you feel God wouldn't be interested or you are ashamed to take Him with you or to include Him? Ask Him how you can acknowledge Him in that area and make Him the source of your strength.

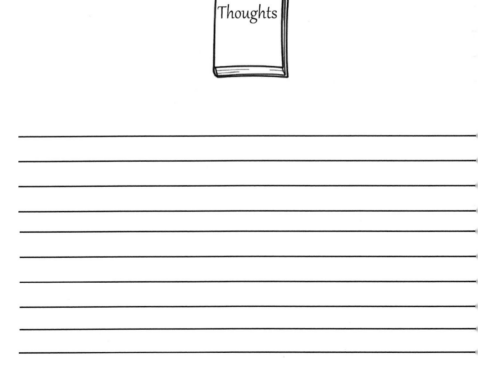

Thoughts

_____

_____

_____

_____

_____

_____

_____

_____

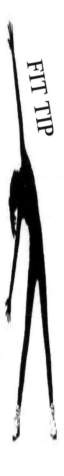

FIT TIP

Balance is the key that can set you free!

Just as you need to draw from the source and strength of God spiritually to bear much fruit, you need to draw from the source and strength of balanced foods nutritionally to be healthy.

One idea of balanced nourishment was summed up by Precision Nutrition with the Handful Rule, an easy way to measure recommended portions of food.

Protein: 2 handfuls for men, 1 for women at every meal

Carbs: 2 handfuls for men, 1 for women at every meal (customize to goals and needs)

Green veggies: At least 1 handful for everyone at every meal

Fruit: 1-2 handfuls per day

Fats: 1-2 handfuls per day

The National Association of Sports Medicine (NASM) measures it a little differently. They recommend:

45%-65% of calories from carbs

20-35% of calories from fat

10-35% of calories from protein

There are apps with calorie counters, such as Fitbit and MyFitnessPal, if you prefer that method. Some prefer the easy Handful Rule because it focuses more on balance and proper portions than counting calories.

Day 32

THE SPIRIT RENEWS

"The Spirit of the Sovereign Lord is on me, because the Lord has anointed me...They will rebuild the ancient ruin and restore the places long devastated; they will renew the ruined cities that have been devastated for generations."

Isaiah 61: 1,4 (NIV)

"...Those who hope in the Lord will renew their strength. They will soar on wings like eagles; they will run and not grow weary, they will walk and not be faint."

Isaiah 40:31 (NIV)

"...And may He be to you a restorer of life and a nourisher of your old age."

Ruth 4:15 (NKJV)

"For as many as are led by the Spirit of God, they are the Sons of God."

Rom. 8:14 (KJV)

Food for Thought

The Spirit of God can renew, redeem, and restore things in your life, even when it seems like you are past the point of no return. Not only does He breathe new life into situations and circumstances, but He renews your strength to go beyond what you thought you could when you rely on Him and allow His Spirit to live in and through you.

To redeem is to recover or buy back. It is to obtain the release or restoration (as from captivity), by paying a ransom. Jesus redeemed us from anything that separated us from God by paying the ransom for us.

In Biblical times, the one who comes to do the redeeming is often a close relative who is in a stronger position and buys back the lost property on behalf of his weaker relative. God is your Father, your relative. You are adopted into His family when you accept His love and sovereignty in your life and heart, and He is able to redeem you.

In the book of Ruth, Boaz was able to redeem Naomi by marrying her daughter-in-law, Ruth. He restored her life and fulfilled her desires with a grandson in her old age. No matter what has happened in your life, it is never too late for God to restore and redeem your circumstance, because He has positioned you as His son or daughter.

Activate

Do you feel like there's an area of your life that needs to be redeemed or set free? Maybe you feel it's too late, or that you're too far gone. Jesus wants to be your Kinsman-Redeemer. Lay your burden at His feet, just as Ruth laid down at Boaz's feet. What do you see when you hide in His wings and allow the wind of His Spirit to take you to higher places?

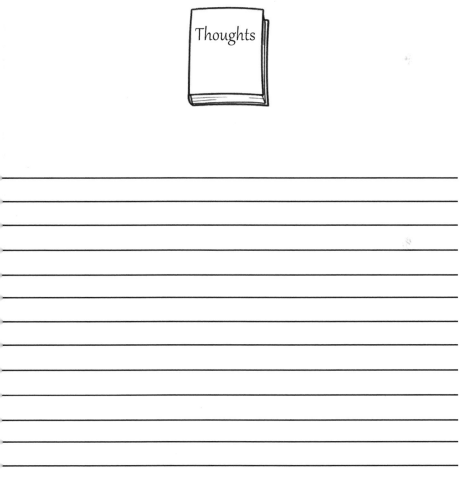

Thoughts

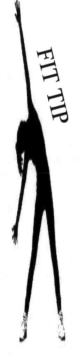

FIT TIP

Stay young at heart by renewing cells that come apart!

A good way to help keep physically young and healthy from the inside-out is by neutralizing free radicals that can accelerate the aging process and contribute to harmful disease. There's a protective coating over your DNA cells called telomeres, which work like plastic shoelace covers keeping them from unraveling. Telomeres protect the cells so they can rejuvenate. However, they shorten as we age, which can be accelerated by stress and unhealthy diet. In order to keep healthy telomeres for proper cell function and antioxidant support, you need a healthy diet and exercise. It's also been proven that the proper combination of Vitamins A, C, E and B12 is beneficial in this process.

There's a supplement with this anti-aging combination listed in the Recommended Resources. (8)

Day 33

FRUIT OF THE SPIRIT IS LOVE

Inspiration

"God is love, and he who abides in love abides in God, and God in Him."

I John 4:16 (NKJV)

"Beloved, let us love one another, for love is of God; and everyone who loves is born of God and knows God."

I John 4:7 (NKJV)

"The fruit of the Spirit is LOVE, joy, peace, longsuffering, kindness, goodness, faithfulness, gentleness, self-control."

Galatians 5:22, 23 (NKJV)

"Love is patient, love is kind. It does not envy, it does not boast, it is not proud. It does not dishonor others, it is not self-seeking, it is not easily angered, it keeps no record of wrongs. Love does not delight in evil but rejoices with the truth. It always protects, always trusts, always hopes, always perseveres.

Love never fails."

I Corinthians 13: 4-8 (NIV)

177

Food for Thought

There is a line in the musical *Les Miserable* that says, "To love another person is to see the face of God." When you love another person, you are seeing God because God is love.

What does God look like? He looks like love. What does love look like...?

Loving another person looks like...being patient with them, being kind to them, honoring them, not turning to anger, being humble and gracious, not having jealousy, putting the other one first, no wishing evil on them, being truthful, protective, trusting, hopeful and persevering.

We have the power to love through God's Spirit, which is love.

When you are filled with the love of God and the Spirit of God lives in you, you produce the fruit of love. Your spirit is led and fed by His Spirit living in you.

In Galatians 5, LOVE is the first and main fruit of the Spirit, from which all the other fruits stem - joy, peace, patience, kindness goodness, faithfulness, gentleness and self-control. Those are the fruits of love. Love is always about relationship over rules. God is love, so He cares more about relationship with you than rules of religion.

Activate

Write out 1 Corinthians 13:4-8, putting God's name in the places it talks about "love". "<u>God</u> is patient, <u>God</u> is kind..." Ask God to fill you with His Spirit of love - especially in those areas you may feel a lack.

Now write it again and put your name "_____ is patient, ____ is kind..." Let God speak to your heart.

Thoughts

_____

_____

_____

_____

_____

_____

_____

_____

_____

_____

_____

_____

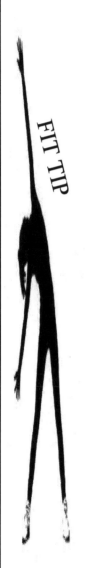

Mood control to keep you whole!

Although love is not necessarily based on a feeling, mood swings and hormones can affect relationships.

Rock Star Syndrome is the let-down usually associated with post-performance. It is caused by the depletion of the hormones serotonin and dopamine, the two primary neurotransmitters in your brain that basically control your emotions, which are produced in mass amounts while performing, causing the euphoric feeling.

Serotonin is regarded by some researchers as the chemical responsible for maintaining mood balance. A deficit of serotonin can lead to depression and lack of being able to solve problems or think clearly. Dopamine is a neurotransmitter that helps control the brain's reward and pleasure centers. Men tend to be low in dopamine, especially when they get older, because testosterone stimulates dopamine. Women tend to be lower in serotonin, which contributes to mood swings. It is primarily found in the GI tract, blood platelets and central nervous system and can be balanced and regulated with supplements. Regulating these neurotransmitters can help with symptoms of ADHD and bipolar disorder.

John Gray, author of *Men Are From Mars, Women Are From Venus,* developed a supplement called Mars Venus Minerals after realizing how important it is to regulate these hormones with nutritionals for balance in a relationship. (9)

Day 34

STRENGTH BY HIS SPIRIT

Inspiration

"Not by might nor by power, but by My Spirit, says the Lord of Hosts."

Zechariah 4:6 (NIV)

"Finally, be strong in the Lord and in his mighty power. Put on the full armor of God, so that you can take your stand against the devil's schemes. For our struggle is not against flesh and blood, but against the rulers, against the authorities, against the powers of this dark world and against the spiritual forces of evil in the heavenly realms. Therefore put on the full armor of God, so that when the day of evil comes, you may be able to stand your ground, and after you have done everything, to stand. Stand firm then, with the belt of truth buckled around your waist, with the breastplate of righteousness in place, and with your feet fitted with the readiness that comes from the gospel of peace. In addition to all this, take up the shield of faith, with which you can extinguish all the flaming arrows of the evil one. Take the helmet of salvation and the sword of the Spirit, which is the word of God.

And pray in the Spirit on all occasions with all kinds of prayers and requests. With this in mind, be alert and always keep on praying for all the Lord's people."

Ephesians 6:10-18 (NIV)

Food for Thought

In Zechariah, God is speaking to the governor of Judah, Zerubbabel, who is ultimately responsible for the rebuilding of the temple. He informs him that the task would not be accomplished through force of an army, nor through the muscular power for physical stamina of the workmen; rather, it would be accomplished by the empowering of the Spirit of God.

In the same way, your temple is rebuilt through His Spirit, you are not fighting just a physical war, but a spiritual one. Your weapons of warfare are truth, righteousness, peace, faith, salvation (God's grace and redemption through Jesus' death and resurrection) God's word, and ultimately prayer - constant communication and open relationship with Him.

It is a spiritual battle, but in order to be strong in your spirit, you can actually put on the armor every day: wrapping truth around your waist, which is associated with your gut or soul; placing righteousness over your chest, which protects your heart; walking in peace, which comes from the gospel of love; holding a shield of faith (God's promises) up against the negative lies that come a you; guarding your mind with a helmet of salvation, the finished work of redemption on the cross; and being ready to fight with the sword of the word of God, which is what Jesus used when He was tempted in the wilderness.

It all culminates in praying in the Spirit - giving it all to God. It is being present with Him, in His presence even to the point of groanings deeper than words. As you do this, the Spirit of God will empower your spirit on a daily basis to rebuild your temple.

Activate

We explored earlier about an area of your temple (or life) that needs to be rebuilt. Ask God to empower you in the Spirit and to show you what that looks like in a practical way on a daily basis. Go through the motions of wrapping the belt of truth around your waist, putting on the breastplate of righteousness, stepping into the boots of peace and walking in love, taking up a shield of faith against lies, putting on a helmet of safety, and drawing your sword of the Spirit. Write how each applies to your situation.

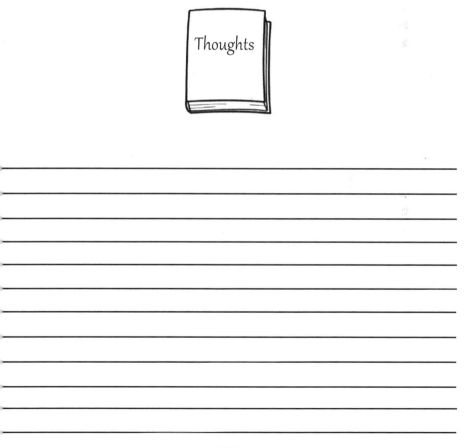

Thoughts

_____

_____

_____

_____

_____

_____

_____

_____

_____

_____

_____

_____

_____

_____

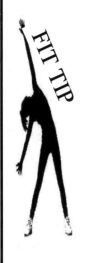

Warfaring Worms

The battle in our body can be against invaders such as parasites. **Intestinal parasites** are organisms that can infect your gastrointestinal tract. They can live throughout the body, but most prefer the intestinal wall. They are usually ingested through undercooked meat or drinking infected water, or they are absorbed through the skin. Consuming sushi or unwashed vegetables can contribute, as well. There are parasite cleanses you can take. Wormwood and black walnut are herbal remedies which can be used to kill parasites and help stimulate digestion.

Day 35

LAW OF THE SPIRIT

"Teacher, which is the greatest commandment in the Law?" Jesus replied: "'Love the Lord your God with all your heart and with all your soul and with all your mind.' This is the first and greatest commandment. And the second is like it: 'Love your neighbor as yourself.' All the Law and the Prophets hang on these two commandments."

Matthew 22:36-40 (NIV)

"You are our letter, written in our hearts,... written not with ink but with the Spirit of the living God, not on tablets of stone but on tablets of human hearts...from God, who also made us adequate as servants of a new covenant, not of the letter but of the Spirit; for the letter kills, but the Spirit gives life."

Corinthians 3:2,3,6 (NASB)

Food for Thought

In the Old Testament the law was given through a written tablet of the Ten Commandments and a lot of rules that went along with it. When Jesus came, the New Covenant was introduced: The Law of the Spirit.

Jesus didn't come to get rid of the Ten Commandments but to fulfill them...with love. If you focus on love (loving the Lord, yourself and your neighbor) they are naturally fulfilled.

When you obey just the letter of the law (rules) over the spirit of it (relationship), you bypass the intent behind it. You never get to the root (love).

Jesus explains how all of the Ten Commandments can be summed up in two commandments of love - love the Lord with everything in you and love your neighbor as yourself. Instead of focusing just on what NOT to do, you are to focus on what TO do. When your heart is focused on LOVING, then the rest falls into place. It is not out of works but out of the grace of love. It is the heart of the law over the letter of the law. The burden of *rules* can kill your spirit but the freedom of *love* can bring your spirit life!

The same is true when you deal with rules or laws of diet or fitness for yourself. Instead of focusing on what you can't have, focus on what is nourishing or healthy. Be grateful you can choose good foods and have the ability and freedom to exercise. Focus on loving God and His creation - YOU - with all of your heart, soul and mind. Then focus on loving yourself by taking care of yourself so that you are freer to love others.

Activate

Instead of writing a list of laws or commandments for yourself (what NOT to do or what NOT to eat), write a list of love rules for yourself. What would be good to do or to eat to feel your best? Ask God to show you His intent and heart for your list.

Thoughts

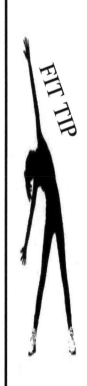

FIT TIP

The One Ingredient Rule

Just as one spiritual law (the law of love) fulfills all the other dos and don'ts, the One Ingredient Rule can take care of the do's and don'ts of nutrition. Look for foods that have just one ingredient - fresh, organic foods are the best. Anything pure and natural. Stay away from processed foods and ones with additives - especially ones that list multiple ingredients that you can't even pronounce!

Diet drinks or foods with aspartame and artificial ingredients actually work against you. Your body doesn't process them correctly and they can cause you to gain weight in the long run. Stick to drinks like water or tea and natural, one-ingredient foods like fruits, vegetables and proteins. If you have to use a sweetener, try to use stevia or small amounts of honey.

Day 36

OPEN SPIRIT

"...the Spirit helps us in our weakness. We do not know what we ought to pray for, but the Spirit Himself intercedes for us through wordless groans."

Romans 8:26 (NIV)

"I will pour out my Spirit on all people. Your sons and daughters will prophesy, your young men will see visions, your old men will dream dreams."

Acts 2:17, Joel 2:28 (NIV)

"As the heavens are higher than the earth, so are my ways higher than your ways and my thoughts higher than your thoughts."

Isaiah 55:9

"I keep asking that...the glorious Father may give you the Spirit of wisdom and revelation, so that you may know Him better. I pray that the eyes of your heart may be enlightened in order that you may know the hope to which He has called you, the riches of His glorious inheritance ... and His incomparably great power..."

Ephesians 1:17-19 (NIV)

Food for Thought

When you are open to the Spirit of God, He gives you revelation and wisdom beyond yourself. His ways and thoughts are higher than yours. He can pour out His Spirit and speak to you and through you in amazing ways. He knows more than you do what you need. He even prays for those things through you when you don't know how to pray for yourself when you release it to Him. He opens your eyes to see the hope and purpose for your life.

"The Spirit of wisdom and revelation" is the unveiling of your heart to receive insight into all God has intended to work in your life, the fullness of who you were created to be.

His ways are higher than yours and He invites you to come up higher with Him. You are His treasure, the apple of His eye, and He wants to bring you higher through the power of His Spirit!

Activate

If you need an answer to something or wisdom in an area, ask God to give you the spirit of revelation to see His ways. Ask God to pour out His Spirit on you - give you His thoughts (or groans!). Write what He shows you or speaks to your heart.

Thoughts

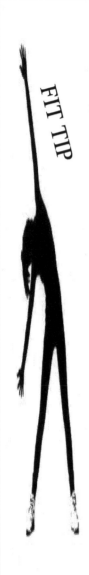

You are the apple of God's eye!

"An apple a day keeps the doctor away."

Loaded with vitamin C, apples support the immune system. The flavonoids in them also have antioxidant effects and can help prevent cardiovascular disease and coronary heart disease.

"An apple a day keeps disease away."

Apples target multiple cancers, such as colon cancer, prostate cancer, and breast cancer. The phenols in apples reduce bad cholesterol and increases good cholesterol.

"An apple a day keeps the memory from going astray."

Apples have phytonutrients that prevent neurodegenerative diseases like Alzheimer's and Parkinson's.

"An apple a day keeps the pounds away."

Apples are a good source of fiber - especially from the skin. One apple has only 70-100 calories and is a good snack

"An apple a day keeps the dentist away!"

The juice of the apples has properties that can kill up to 80% of bacteria which helps eliminate tooth decay.

Day 37

SPIRIT TO SPIRIT

'But when He, the Spirit of Truth, comes, He will guide you into all truth. He will not speak on his own; He will speak only what He hears, and He will tell you what is yet to come."

John 16:13 (NIV)

'But the Helper, the Holy Spirit, whom the Father will send in My name, He will teach you all things, and bring to your remembrance all things that I said to you."

John 14:26 (NKJV)

"Whether you turn to the right or to the left, your ears will hear a voice behind you, saying, "This is the way; walk in it." Isaiah 30:21 (NIV)

"There is now no condemnation for those who are in Christ Jesus, because...the law of the Spirit of life has set me free."

Romans 8:1-2 (NIV)

Food for Thought

Your spirit will recognize and resonate with the Spirit of God the more you align yourself with His truth. He will bring to remembrance His Word. He is called "The Helper". He will counsel you and guide you. Your spirit can sense when He is speaking just as a sheep hears his shepherd, you can hear His voice guiding you or nudging you if you are going off the path.

What does His voice sound like? It can be a still small voice, as we discussed in the two-way journaling. Or it can be *knowing* in your spirit. Or it can come through someone else or through a sign. But it always lines up with the truth of His Word and character.

His voice does not *condemn* - it may point out where you are missing the mark, but only to draw you back to Himself out of love. Satan is known as the accuser. God is the lover of our hearts.

> *"For God did not send His Son into the world to condemn the world, but that the world, through Him, might be saved."*
>
> *John 3:17 (NKJV)*

Activate

If you are needing counsel in an area or direction, ask God to speak to you through His Spirit. Ask Him the question and wait for the answer. Wait for His voice to speak to your spirit and write what you hear.

Thoughts

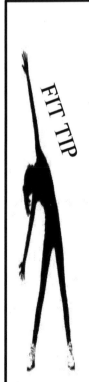

FIT TIP

Lengthen your range!

Just as you need to be flexible in allowing the Spirit to speak to you as a Helper to increase spiritual awareness and truth, flexibility training (stretching) is an essential component to a full-workout program because it increases range of movement in the joints,, improves circulation (which increases energy levels), promotes better posture, and is an excellent method for treating back pain. Regular flexibility workouts can also reduce muscle tension and relieve stress. Plus, stretching just feels good, which is as good for our psyche as it is for our bodies.

A great form of stretching is resistance stretching. One of the best ways to do this is on a Pilates reformer, where you are strengthening and lengthening at the same time. If you don't have access to that, you can use an exercise band following a video or online demonstration.

Day 38

FEEDING THE SPIRIT

Inspiration

'Those who live according to the flesh set their minds on the things of the flesh, but those who live according to the Spirit, the things of the Spirit... But if the Spirit of Him who raised Jesus from the dead dwells in you, He who raised Christ from the dead will also give life to your mortal bodies through His Spirit who dwells in you.'

Romans. 8: 2,5,11 (NKJV)

'But He said to them, 'I have food to eat of which you do not know.' Therefore the disciples said to one another, 'Has anyone brought Him anything to eat?' Jesus said to them, 'My food is to do the will of Him who sent Me, and to finish His work.'''

John 4:32-34 (NKJV)

'..Is not life more than food?'

Matthew 6:25 (NKJV)

You are fed by more than just food. Walking in purpose feeds your spirit. When you focus on the things you feel called to do and what you were created for, God's will for your life, He provides for and fulfills you.

There's nothing wrong with enjoying good food, but sometimes it becomes an idol when you just live to eat or are even obsessed with diet; living not to eat! When you have a focus on God's will for your life - doing what He has created you for - then that becomes the food that sustains you. Putting it in proper perspective and priority can keep your life centered and balanced.

Activate

Ask God to show you what His will or work is in you - what is the food He wants you to feed on or focus on? What would be on your plate? Ask Him for a vision for your life if you are not seeing one.

Thoughts

_____

_____

_____

What are you feeding?

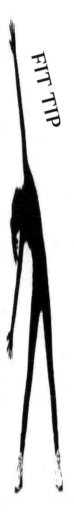

FIT TIP

Although there is a physiological hunger, there are many other reasons people eat. Nutritional hunger is a physical response to lack of fuel, where your blood sugar plunges, which can make you irritable, weak, and shaky. It can create headaches and hunger pangs. It is important to fuel your body with good energy at that point with at least a healthy snack.

However, other ways you may be hungering "could be "emotional or spiritual. These hungers cannot be filled with food. Empty space may be masked as hunger for food, especially these days with so much constant stimulation. You may need to ask yourself what it is you are actually hungering for. Sometimes, you can grab food out of boredom or emotions such as anger, sadness, depression or irritability. Other times, it may be from procrastination or mindless eating out of distraction (while watching TV, for example). PMS or hormones can mask cravings for sweets as hunger. Try grabbing a healthier alternative, such as a piece of dark chocolate or nuts. Organic popcorn made with coconut oil is a healthy, fulfilling snack.

A couple of other good snacks that can keep your metabolism going and satisfy cravings, especially during fasting days, are listed in the Recommended Resources (10).

Day 39

FULLNESS OF THE SPIRIT

Inspiration

'Those who are led by the Spirit of God are sons of God...the Spirit you received brought about your adoption to sonship. And by Him we cry, "Abba, Father."

Romans 8:14,15 (NIV)

'I will not leave you as orphans; I will come to you." John 14:18 (NIV)

"God has said, 'Never will I leave you; never will I forsake you.'"

Hebrews 13:5 (NIV)

'The thief does not come except to steal, and to kill, and to destroy. I have come that they may have life, and that they may have it more abundantly."

John 10:10 (NKJV)

"Whoever believes in me, as scripture has said, rivers of living water will flow from within them."

John 7:38 (NIV)

Food for Thought

Jesus broke the chains of death and destruction so that you could have life to the fullest as a child of God. In His Kingdom abundance supersedes scarcity. There is always enough to go around.

When you understand your identity, it helps your perception and self-image. You are a child of God. You are not an orphan. Orphans operate out of a spirit of scarcity because they never know if there will be enough to go around. God says there is always enough. Orphans feel like they have to fight for themselves and defend what they have. They don't trust that someone will care for them so they operate out of self-preservation.

Sometimes when you diet or try to restrict yourself, you take on the orphan mentality. You feel like you are missing out and you'll never be able to eat that again, so you just do the opposite and it starts a vicious cycle. Recognize that the thief is trying to steal your joy and destroy you through guilt or feeling you have to take care of yourself or fend for yourself as if you are an orphan. He wants to rob your spirit from being free to step into the abundant life God has for you. God said that He will take care of you as His child and that He will never leave or forsake you.

You were created for fullness. When you stop operating out of a spirit of scarcity and allow His spirit to overwhelm you, then rivers of living water will flow in and through you.

You were created for abundance!

Activate

s there an area where you feel you are operating in scarcity and not abundance? Perhaps it's like looking through a big picture window where everyone is laughing and eating a feast at a long table by the fireplace and you are left outside in the cold. Try stepping into the room. "Knock and the door will be opened to you." Matthew 7:7 (NIV). Ask God to show you the treasures and feast He has for you as His child.

f you knew you would always be loved fully and unconditionally and would be provided for, how would you live? Ask God to show you how you can live that way today and sit at that table. He said He would supply ALL your needs according to His riches in glory. Philippians 4:19)

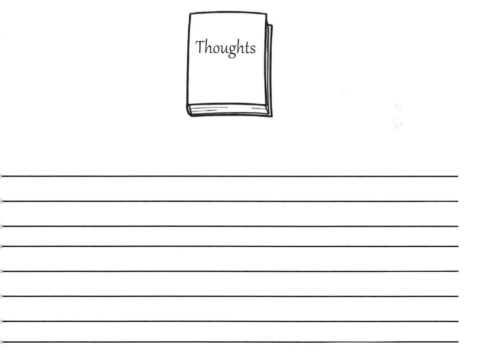

Thoughts

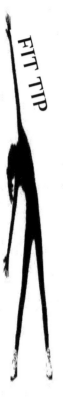

FIT TIP

"When life gives you lemons, make lemonade"!

You may feel like you've been given lemons in life, yet it is sometimes the lemons that create character, balance and even creativity in your life.

Physically, lemons are sour, but they actually can create balance in your body with PH levels, and have many benefits. Because of the potassium, vitamins C, B6, A, and E, folate, niacin, thiamin, riboflavin, pantothenic acid, copper, calcium, zinc, phosphorus, magnesium, antioxidants, and iron in them, they can help in hydration, glowing skin, enhanced immunities and diminishing inflammation. They can also be a beneficial antibacterial and antiviral support and help with digestion. They have a neutralizing effect on stomach acid to ease digestion and prevent inflammation and can flush toxins.

That's why it is recommended to have a glass of lemon water when you first wake up. Lemons are even known to freshen breath, which is a good reason to drink the lemon water served at a restaurant, especially on a date!

Day 40

GOD'S WHOLE, HOLY HEART FOR YOU

Inspiration

"For I am convinced that neither death nor life, neither angels nor demons, neither the present nor the future, nor any powers, neither height nor depth, nor anything else in all creation, will be able to separate us from the love of God that is in Christ Jesus our Lord."

Romans 8:38-39 (NIV)

"I pray "that He would grant you, according to the riches of His glory, to be strengthened with might through His Spirit in the inner man, that Christ may dwell in your hearts through faith; that you, being rooted and grounded in love, may be able to comprehend with all the saints what is the width and length and depth and height— to know the love of Christ which passes knowledge; that you may be filled with all the fullness of God."

Ephesians 3:16-19 (NKJV)

"Now to Him who is able to do exceedingly abundantly above all that we ask or think, according to the power that works in us, to Him be glory in the church by Christ Jesus to all generations, forever and ever. Amen."

Ephesians 3:20-21(NKJV)

Food for Thought

God's love for you can never be pulled away. It is unconditiona[l] and immeasurable. He wants you to be whole in mind, body, sou[l] and spirit and to be holy, which simply means *set apart o[r] separate* from anything that separates you from Him and from Hi[s] love. He wants you to be standing in the joy, love and authorit[y] given to you through Jesus because of God's great love and grac[e] toward you.

God's desire is that you be filled up with His love and that yo[u] would begin to grasp the goodness and faithfulness of His hear[t] toward you in every way. He wants to fill you beyond what yo[u] could ask or imagine and pour His love in and through you i[n] every area of your life so that it overflows onto others. His desir[e] is that your mind, body soul and spirit be Whole and Holy, full[y] Fit and fully Free!

Activate

Is there anything that you feel separates you from the love of God? Ask God to help you *separate* from it!

Ask God to speak to your heart and show you His unconditional, immeasurable love for you. Maybe just ask the question, "Do you love me?"

Invite Him to do exceedingly, abundantly beyond what you could ask or imagine in your life!

Thoughts

_____

_____

_____

_____

_____

_____

_____

_____

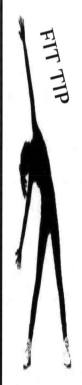

FIT TIP

Creating a lifestyle of health and freedom!

Nutrition and exercise are not a diet and fitness program, but a lifestyle. The key is balance and grace. Eating "fit" foods (nutritional) on a daily basis can alter your life and create habits of health and wellness. Allowing yourself the occasional "free" food (fun food, like dark chocolate) keeps the variety and keeps you out of bondage. Staying away from "fake" food (processed, refined and artificial food) can keep you from the stuff that is actually harmful to you.

Exercise to stay fit, but allow yourself the joy and freedom within that!

It is this balance of discipline and grace
    While you are running your life's race
    With the vision to be the best YOU can be
        That will keep you wHoly Fit and wHoly Free!

Recommended Resources

These are the recommendations mentioned throughout the Fit Tips relating to specific areas of health.

1. IsaLean Pro Shake
2. Brain Boost and Renewal
3. Cleanse For Life (Plus 30 Day Cleanse Program)
4. Essentials (for Women or for Men)
5. Ionix Supreme
6. Kangen Water (Leonslivingwater.com)
7. Sleep Support and Renewal
8. Genesis B
9. Mars Venus Minerals (for Women or for Men)
10. IsaDelight Chocolate Snacks, and Amped Protein Bar

You can find these at: www.wHolyFitwHolyFree.Isagenix.com.

For even more information, or to get a personal assessment for reaching your quality of life potential, go to www.SusanSilvestri.com.

To book a life-empowering message for your group, contact Sue@SusanSilvestri.com.

Recommended Reading

Your Third Brain
Marco Ruggiero MD and Peter Greenlaw

The TDOS Syndrome
Peter Greenlaw

The Mars and Venus Diet & Exercise Solution
John Gray, PHD

Translating God and God Secrets
Shawn Bolz

Birthing The Miraculous and There is Always Enough
Heidi Baker

4 Keys To Hearing God's Voice
Mark Virkler
http://www.cwgministries.org/Four-Keys-to-Hearing-Gods-Voice

About the Author

Susan Silvestri is founder and keynote speaker of Women of Worth, A Creative Encounter, where she uses her book, *wHoly Fit, wHoly Free,* to encourage and activate women to hear God's voice for themselves through creativity. This experience includes two-way journaling and movement (dance) and often incorporates painting, worship, film and comedy. It empowers women to fill the mind, body, soul and spirit with the truth of who God says they are and develop a healthy self-image through creative activations.

To book a creative seminar, contact Susan Silvestri at Sue@SusanSilvestri.com.

You can also visit her website at www.SusanSilvestri.com.

Made in the USA
San Bernardino, CA
27 September 2018